12WBT
Low-carb
SOLUTION

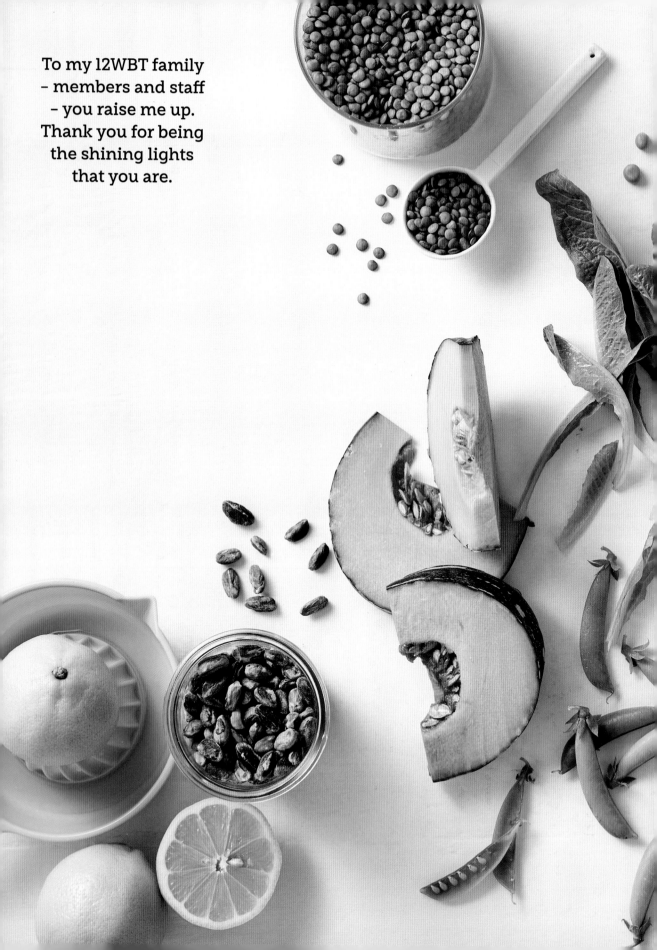

To my 12WBT family
– members and staff
– you raise me up.
Thank you for being
the shining lights
that you are.

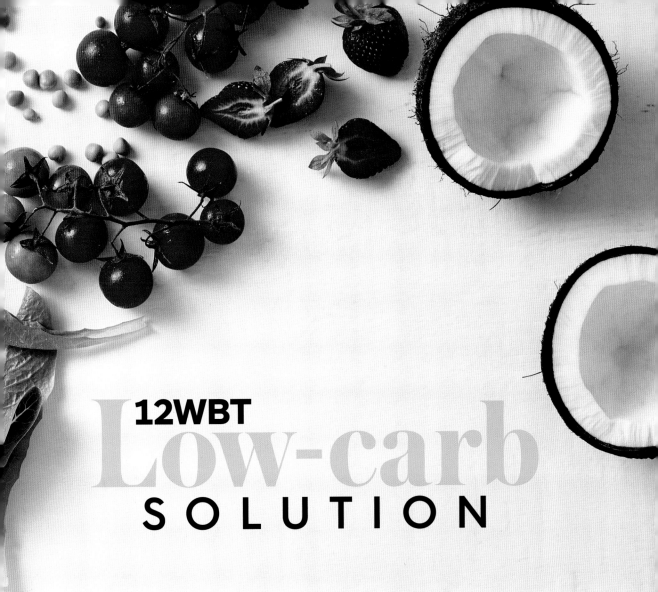

12WBT
Low-carb
SOLUTION

Michelle
Bridges

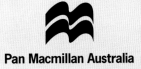

Pan Macmillan Australia

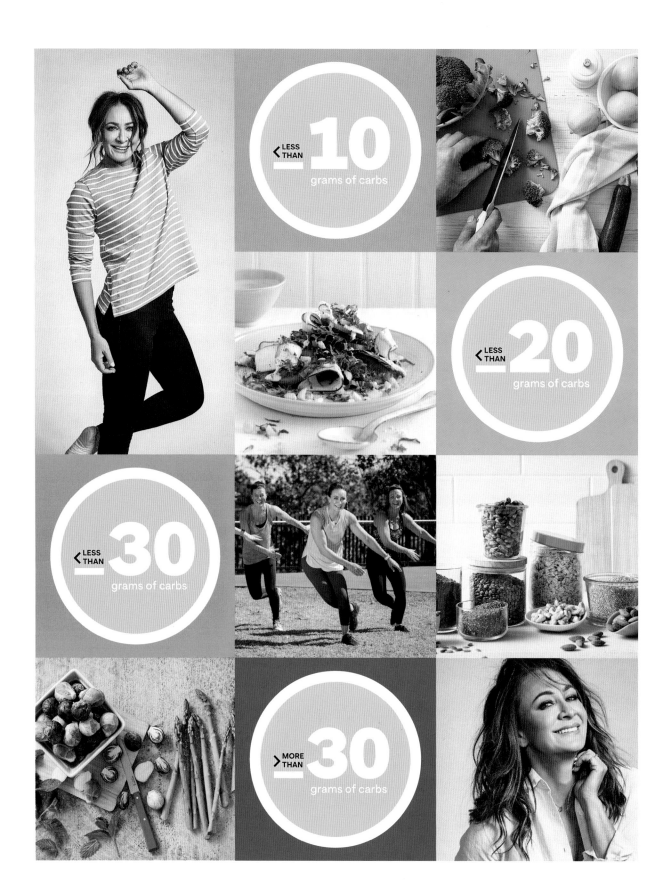

Contents

Introduction 6

PART ONE
The low-carb solution

Carbohydrates 101 12

Carb overload and the road to ill-health 14

Carbs and gut health 18

What is low-carb? 20

My favourite smart carbs 24

Simple carb swaps 26

My day on a plate 28

The exercise bit 32

Snacks and exercise 36

Four low-carb meal plans 45

PART TWO
The recipes

Less than 10 grams of carbs 63

Less than 20 grams of carbs 101

Less than 30 grams of carbs 161

More than 30 grams of carbs 211

Conversion chart 252

Michelle's story 253

Acknowledgements 253

Index 254

Introduction

I've spent the best part of three decades working to help people understand how the food they eat and the exercise they do affects their physical and mental wellbeing — inspiring them to become the best version of themselves that they can be. It's an awesome job and a passion that began early for me.

I remember in Year 8 I noticed there were kids at my school who didn't join in with any team games and instead hung around smoking cigarettes. It got me thinking. Clearly these kids didn't feel comfortable playing organised sports — I could understand that, we're all different — but I felt they were missing out. By this stage I'd already been doing team sports for years and I knew how exercise could boost my mood, help me concentrate and build my self-confidence, so I asked the school principal if I could teach fitness classes. She said yes and I was beyond delighted. Every week, I blasted my music and a small group of us leapt around doing grapevines, squat jumps and push-ups. I mention this because I honestly wanted to help those kids, just as I have wanted to help every brave contestant on *The Biggest Loser*, every client I have trained, and every open-hearted person who has enrolled in my 12WBT program.

But the sad fact is that we still aren't doing so well on our 'Health Report Card'. Here's a snapshot of all the recent data I could get my hands on. This stuff rips my heart out:

* Almost two-thirds (63 per cent) of Australians aged 18 and over, and more than one-quarter (28 per cent) of children aged 5–17 are overweight or obese, putting them at risk of high blood pressure, cardiovascular disease, diabetes and arthritis.
* 1 in 3 Australian adults has high blood pressure.
* Cardiovascular disease kills 1 Australian every 12 minutes. This is the time it takes me to have a shower, towel down and get dressed — a truly overwhelming thought.
* 1 in 20 Australians had diabetes in 2017–18, with an average of 291 new people registering with the National Diabetes Scheme every single day.
* 1 in 5 Australians aged 16–85 will also experience mental illness in any given year, with suicide being the leading cause of death for those aged 25–44.

I want to help change this. I don't want YOU to become part of these stats. In my first book, *Crunch Time*, I urged readers to choose foods that were as close to their natural state as possible and to feel empowered by making these choices. Yes we live in an obesogenic environment (fast food at every turn, our supermarkets packed to the rafters with processed food), but ultimately we are in charge of what we load into our shopping bags. The problem is that we are literally bombarded with constantly changing information about what, when and how we should eat and drink. Should we ditch gluten? Stop eating red meat? What about fasting? And do probiotics really help? It's no wonder many of us give up in frustration.

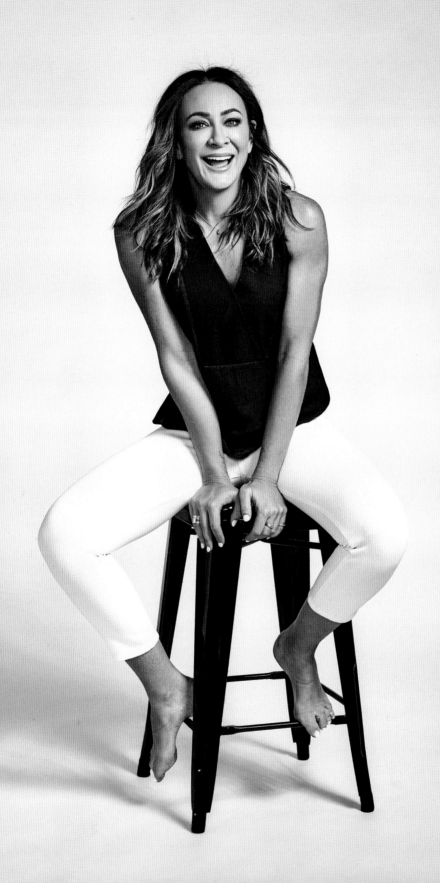

I've always tried to avoid using the word 'diet' when explaining my nutrition principles – it's a word with way too much baggage – but I have always advocated eating a moderate amount of protein, a small amount of good-quality fat, lots of leafy greens and the right carbs. And this just so happens to correlate with what many are now calling a 'low-carb' approach to eating. Notice I said 'low carb', not 'no carb'. I'm not going to tell you that carbs alone are killing us, no way, but I reckon we can do so much better when it comes to choosing the right carbs in the right amounts, which is why I wrote this book.

My mission is to show you that low-carb eating is easy, fun and tastes amazing. Even better, it has incredible health benefits for your blood sugar level, metabolism, gut and brain. First I'll explain the different types of carbs and how they impact the body. No doubt you'll already know that sugary drinks, lollies and biscuits have got to be kicked to the kerb if you're serious about your health. But I also want to show you why whole plant foods are the best choice not only for total body health, but also mental wellbeing.

However, I'm not going to lie to you. If you're used to eating pastries, pasta and white bread or lots of sugar, dialling down the carbs is not going to be easy. That's why I've included 120 of my 12WBT low-carb recipes, each with the right balance of carbs, protein and fats to keep you feeling full and give you sustained energy throughout the day. I've also provided four dietitian-approved meal plans to help you get started. Each features a creative use of leftovers (so you're not cooking from scratch every day – who has time for that?!) and I also outline simple ingredient swaps (for particular tastes) and carb boosters for when you need to dial up the energy intake for hungry teenagers, manual workers or sport-loving humans. Think of the meal plans as your training wheels – soon enough you won't need them any more and can confidently go it alone.

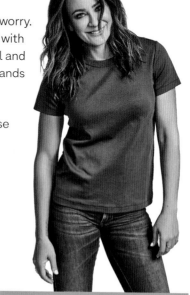

If you're not familiar with my 12WBT program, don't worry. All you need to know is that good nutrition coupled with exercise is a powerful path back to positive physical and mental health. I've seen it change the lives of thousands of my 12WBTers and personal training clients.

Just by being smart about the (low) carbs you choose every day means you'll:

√ Reduce your blood sugar level.
√ Reduce your hunger.
√ Store less fat.
√ Improve your gut health.
√ Improve your brain function.
√ Improve your mental health.

But don't just take my word for it!

Rachel

I thought I knew all there was to know about food, lifestyle and nutrition. How wrong I was! 12WBT gave me the knowledge I needed around wholesome nutrition to fuel my body for not just exercise, but for life!

Samantha

This has been the only program that has worked where I can see it as a lifestyle and not a quick fix, counting the days till I can eat carbs, sugar or whatever it was that I had to give up! The nutrition programs are simple to follow and sustainable for long-term health.

Sonia

I can't express how grateful I am for such a well-balanced, easy-to-follow, well-structured program. My desire for a healthier and fitter me outweighed my desire to eat junk food, which was a massive turning point halfway through the program. It was because I never felt deprived or hungry as I was nourishing my body regularly with delicious, simple-to-prepare meals! I am now a girl living her best life!

Anna

There probably isn't a diet plan I haven't tried! You lose weight on most of them but they are so hard to stick to that you fall off the wagon before long. Then a few years ago I discovered 12WBT and I never looked back. What I loved most about 12WBT was it was real food that the whole family could enjoy, which meant we could all eat the same thing together, and the meals were so easy to prepare. The weekly meal plans meant I didn't have to spend time thinking about what to eat for the week and the amazing shopping lists meant I didn't have to spend hours writing out shopping lists. A few clicks and it was done. The best part was it encouraged us as a family to try new recipes, even ones we didn't think we would like that actually ended up being some of our favourites. The step-by-step recipes were also simple to follow, even for someone like me that can't cook!

Hila

With this program, and the variety of recipes and meal plans, I didn't feel I had to give up on anything, just reshape portions and regularity [of meals]. I feel so good now that I am going to keep my new habits and my 'new me' and enjoy life.

PART ONE

The low-carb solution

Carbohydrates 101

Forgive the high school science lesson, but once you understand how the food you eat affects your body, I guarantee you will be even more determined to make better food choices. Many of my 12WBTers say exactly that (see Nerida's story on page 31).

Like proteins and fats, carbs are one of the three macronutrients that our bodies need to stay healthy and strong. (They're called 'macro' because we need them in relatively large amounts compared to the micronutrients – vitamins, minerals and polyphenols – which are critical for helping the macros do their job.)

Carbohydrates supply the body with glucose, the preferred fuel for our brain, kidneys and red blood cells, and the fuel we use when we start to exercise. If we don't eat enough carbs, our muscles, lungs and heart will burn fat for fuel (this is the essence of the keto diet, see page 20) and if we run out of fat, the body must break down protein (aka muscle) to make the glucose it needs.

All plant foods contain carbs (vegetables, fruit, grains, nuts, seeds and legumes) as do milk and dairy products. There are no carbs in meat, poultry, fish and seafood and little to none in eggs. Instead, these are rich in the amino acids necessary to build and repair body tissue, and to make the enzymes and hormones that facilitate the bazillion chemical reactions that keep us alive.

SIMPLE AND COMPLEX CARBS

You may have heard carbs described as 'simple' or 'complex', though this division is becoming less useful the more we understand about how carbs influence both our metabolic and gut health.

Carbohydrates are made up of molecules of **carb**on, **o**xygen and **hyd**rogen (hence the name) which group together in different ways to make saccharides (from the Latin word for sugar). The simplest carbs are called monosaccharides, and include glucose, fructose and galactose (there are many more). These guys are rarely found on their own in nature and instead form the building blocks for bigger carbs. When two monosaccharides react, they make disaccharides such as sucrose (a combo of glucose and fructose) and lactose (a combo of glucose and galactose). All of these break down rapidly in the body to give us an instant energy hit, which is why they're often lumped together and called 'simple sugars' (and usually have names ending in 'ose'). They're found naturally in honey, milk and fruit and are also extracted from plants such as sugar cane, sugar beets, corn and the sap of maple trees.

Polysaccharides are formed from long chains of monosaccharides, and include starch and cellulose. Starch is a plant's energy store and exists in two forms: amylose (which is soluble and therefore digestible for humans) and amylopectin (which is not). Plants need cellulose to strengthen cell walls and provide structure during growth. Humans can't digest cellulose (we lack the enzyme needed to break it down), but it's an important source of fibre.

Starch and cellulose are found in fruits, veggies (cellulose especially in the stems and skins),

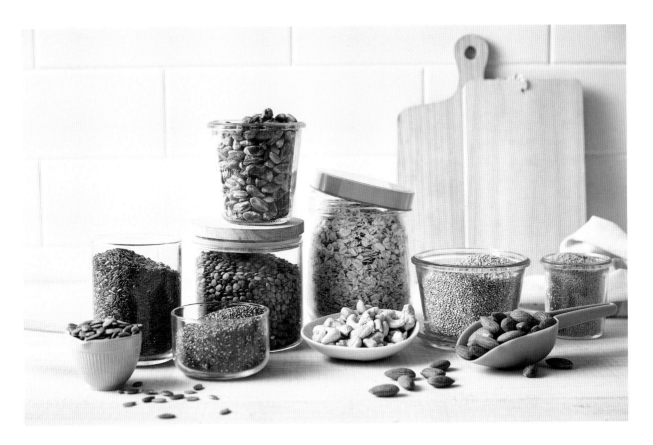

nuts, seeds, beans, lentils, peas and grains such as wheat, oats, rice, quinoa and buckwheat.

WHAT HAPPENS WHEN WE EAT CARBS?

When we eat sugars and digestible starches, amylase (an enzyme in our saliva) immediately begins breaking them down so that by the time they reach the gut, they're ready to be absorbed into the bloodstream as glucose. Indigestible starches and cellulose will pass straight through to the large intestine to help bulk stools and keep us regular, as well as feed our army of friendly gut bacteria.

In order to get the glucose into our cells, the pancreas releases insulin, a hormone that signals cells to take it up. Some of our cells will use the glucose immediately, while liver and muscle cells store it as glycogen (the name for clusters of glucose molecules) ready to be used later. However, our muscles and liver have a limit on how much glycogen they can store

(usually only enough for one day), and when that limit is reached, the excess is stored as fat. Eating more carbs than we need, day after day, and doing very little exercise, is a one-way street to weight gain and disease.

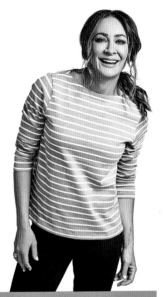

Counting carbs is of no benefit without consideration of their quality . . . Put simply, we must choose carbs as they exist in nature.

Carb overload and the road to ill-health

As I mentioned in the intro, carbs are not the enemy. They are an important energy source and also supply us with the vitamins, minerals and polyphenols (antioxidant plant compounds) that keep all our body systems functioning properly.

But that only applies if we are eating carbs that are close to their natural state: legumes, whole grains, nuts, seeds, veggies and fruit. If we're chowing down on foods made from refined flour and sugar, and not exercising, we face a whole range of avoidable health problems. Here's a rough explanation of how things go.

SUGAR, INSULIN RESISTANCE AND TYPE 2 DIABETES

If we eat a lot of sugar in one hit, we have what's called an insulin spike, where our pancreas releases a stack of insulin to help our cells take up the excess glucose. When this happens day after day, our cells can eventually become desensitised ('resistant') to insulin and stop responding as they should. This leaves us with elevated blood sugar levels, forcing our pancreas to release more and more insulin to try to get those levels down.

Chronically elevated insulin does several things:

* It signals more fat to be stored (part of the reason we keep gaining weight).
* It interferes with the proper signalling of our appetite hormones.
* It stops the thyroid working properly.
* It damages the lining of our blood vessels.
* It increases our risk of developing type 2 diabetes.

Type 2 diabetes develops when there is too much glucose in the bloodstream, which over time can severely damage the eyes, kidneys and nerves, leading to blindness, kidney failure, ulcers and limb amputations. (Not to be confused with type 1 diabetes, which is an autoimmune condition where sufferers require daily insulin injections. About 5 per cent of diabetics have this type.) Having type 2 diabetes also doubles the risk of heart attack and stroke. This is because chronic high blood glucose can damage the heart and also lead to more fatty deposits in the blood vessel walls.

Diabetes Australia reports that one person is diagnosed with diabetes every five minutes, and while genes have a role to play, carrying excess fat is the greatest risk factor (check out the box on the opposite page). Yet unlike genetics, this is a *modifiable* risk factor. And there is increasing evidence that even a modest amount of weight loss can reduce the risk of diabetes and the inevitable heart disease that follows. You see, diabetes itself doesn't kill people.

A 2016 study of 40 obese men and women in England showed that reducing their weight by just 5 per cent improved their blood pressure, circulating triglycerides and blood sugar levels, which are all risk factors for diabetes and heart disease. Losing 10 per cent of their weight showed even more improvements.

HOW MUCH SUGAR DO WE 'NEED'?

In 2015, the World Health Organization recommended that free sugars ('monosaccharides and disaccharides added to foods and beverages by the manufacturer, cook or consumer, and sugars naturally present in honey, syrups, fruit juices and fruit juice concentrates') should make up less than 10 per cent of our total energy intake. So, if we're taking in 1600–1800 calories per day, then the total amount of extra sugar in our diets should be around 8–9 teaspoons per day. To me, even that seems a lot, especially when we can get all the glucose we need from the starches in grains and veggies. And in fact, some countries (e.g. the UK) are advising that free sugars should make up no more than 5 per cent of our total energy intake.

As you know from my previous books, and my 12WBT program, I rarely add sugar to any of my recipes, apart from the occasional teaspoon of brown sugar or honey or a date here and there (dried fruit is very high in sugar). I may also use a small amount of good-quality oyster sauce or chilli sauce, but I always check the labels to make sure they don't contain extra sugars in the form of corn starch, maltose, dextrose etc.

Soft drinks and cordials are definitely out (a single can contains 7½ teaspoons of sugar – that's close to your daily quota right there) and I've always banged on about dodging biscuits, cakes, pastries and the like, not only because they are usually packed with sugar, but also because they're nearly always made with refined white flour.

You see, refined flour is made from grains (most often wheat, but also rye and barley) that have been stripped of their husk, bran and germ to increase shelf life. (The bran and germ contain proteins and oils that can denature when exposed to air and heat, which is why it's best to store your whole-grain flour in the fridge or freezer.) White flour is basically starch, which as you now know, is rapidly converted to glucose in the body. When we constantly overload the body with too much sugar and starch, it not only

Obesity and diabetes

In 2017–18 the Australian Bureau of Statistics National Health Survey found that adults aged 18 years and over who were obese were almost five times as likely as those who were of normal weight to have type 2 diabetes (9.8 per cent compared to 2.0 per cent). Similarly, adults who were overweight were more than twice as likely to have type 2 diabetes (4.6 per cent compared to 2.0 per cent) than adults of a normal weight.

However, not all people who develop diabetes are overweight or obese. This is where the 'body mass index' scale (BMI) used to classify people's weight can be misleading, especially for people in the overweight category. ('Normal weight' is a BMI of 18.5 to 24.9; 'overweight' is 25 to 29.9 and 'obese' is 30 or greater.) The problem is that BMI does not take into account the amount of body fat a person carries, or where it is carried.

Researchers have found that if you carry a lot of fat around your waist (called visceral fat), it increases your risk of suffering a heart attack, stroke or other cardiovascular disease, even if your BMI is normal. In one 2019 study of post-menopausal women published in the *European Heart Journal*, investigators found that women with the highest percentage of fat stored around their middles and trunks and the lowest around their legs had more than three times the risk of cardiovascular disease than women with the reverse (a low percentage of fat around their middles and a higher percentage of fat around the legs).

The take-home message? Make sure your doctor or health professional not only looks at your BMI, but also your waist measurement.

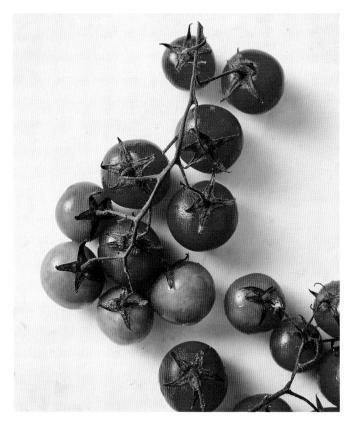

FRUCTOSE AND FATTY LIVER

Not all simple sugars are metabolised in the same way. While glucose can be used by every cell in the body, only liver cells can take up fructose. So when we eat a lot of fructose in one go (remember cane sugar is 50 per cent fructose), it goes straight to the liver via the portal vein where some is converted to glucose and glycogen but most is immediately converted to fat.

Scientists believe this metabolic variation evolved because our hunter-gatherer ancestors only occasionally found honey, berries and other fruits. So, to make the best use of this rare energy source, they were able to eat their fill and store it immediately. In other words, we didn't evolve a 'full' switch that told our bodies we'd had enough fructose. This means we can eat loads of fructose-containing foods without feeling full, which is why we can drink a litre of fruit juice, but would struggle to drink a litre of milk.

Researchers have found that high intakes of fructose (in the form of sucrose or high-fructose corn syrup) can rapidly induce fat accumulation in the liver, and that reducing fructose can reverse it. Unchecked high consumption can result in non-alcoholic fatty liver disease (NAFLD), where liver cells start to die off, leaving scar tissue (fibrosis) that reduces liver function. Not surprisingly, NAFLD is strongly associated with obesity, insulin resistance and metabolic syndrome (see box on the opposite page).

The good news is that whole fruits are less likely to induce metabolic syndrome due to their lower fructose content (compared to a soft drink) and also because they contain vitamins and polyphenols (compounds that give plants their colour and flavour) that act as antioxidants in the body.

leads to weight gain but also starts to mess with our metabolism, putting us at risk of developing insulin resistance and type 2 diabetes.

Flours and cereals made from whole grains, on the other hand, take longer to digest, slowing the release of glucose into the bloodstream. Plus the fibrous bran is good for the bowel. More on that a bit later.

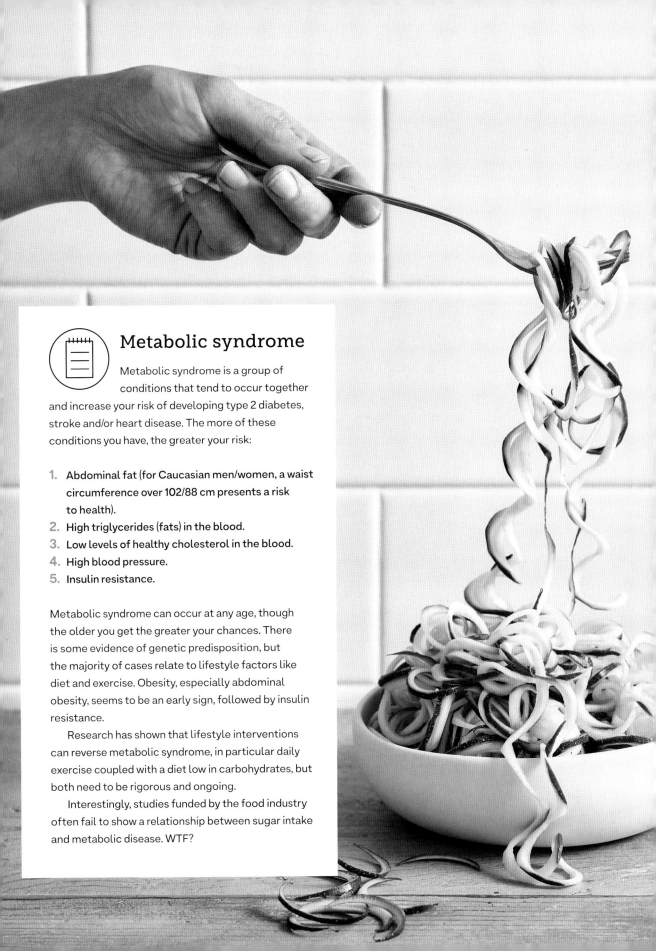

Metabolic syndrome

Metabolic syndrome is a group of conditions that tend to occur together and increase your risk of developing type 2 diabetes, stroke and/or heart disease. The more of these conditions you have, the greater your risk:

1. Abdominal fat (for Caucasian men/women, a waist circumference over 102/88 cm presents a risk to health).
2. High triglycerides (fats) in the blood.
3. Low levels of healthy cholesterol in the blood.
4. High blood pressure.
5. Insulin resistance.

Metabolic syndrome can occur at any age, though the older you get the greater your chances. There is some evidence of genetic predisposition, but the majority of cases relate to lifestyle factors like diet and exercise. Obesity, especially abdominal obesity, seems to be an early sign, followed by insulin resistance.

Research has shown that lifestyle interventions can reverse metabolic syndrome, in particular daily exercise coupled with a diet low in carbohydrates, but both need to be rigorous and ongoing.

Interestingly, studies funded by the food industry often fail to show a relationship between sugar intake and metabolic disease. WTF?

Carbs and gut health

As we saw earlier, plants contain fibre (cellulose and starches) that feed the billions of bacteria (the microbiome) that live in our gut, particularly our colons. These microbes basically ferment the carbs, producing short-chain fatty acids (butyrate, propionate and acetate) as a by-product.

Butyrate is especially important as it provides fuel for the epithelial cells of our large intestine, enhancing gut wall integrity and immune function. You see, close to 70 per cent of our immune system is housed in our gastrointestinal tract (all those immune cells such as macrophages and T-cells), which is why it is so important to keep the lining healthy.

Scientists are still busy identifying different species in the microbiome and their specific roles, but they do know that diversity is a key factor in gut health and therefore immune function. Studies have found that having fewer bacterial species is a common feature of obesity, bowel disease, depression and other inflammatory conditions.

So what's the best way to encourage a diverse microbiome? To feed our little helpers the fibre they love from as many different kinds of veggies, fruit, legumes and whole grains as we can. This is why I've included 'Meatless Mondays' in the meal plans to help you focus on getting some nourishing and valuable prebiotic legumes and veggies into your diet.

FIBRE

Dietary fibre has traditionally been classified as either insoluble (roughage) or soluble (readily fermented by gut bacteria). But this classification system doesn't work for resistant starch, which is why it gets a heading of its own.

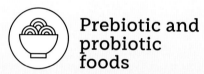

Prebiotic and probiotic foods

Prebiotic foods (namely legumes, whole grains, fruit and veg) feed the microbes that are already living in your gut, which we know has important flow-on effects for digestion and immune function.

Probiotic foods (such as yoghurt, kefir, kimchi, kombucha and sauerkraut) actually contain living bacterial species (such as Lactobacillus), which add to our resident population of beneficial microbes.

Importantly, whether we feed them or ingest them, the bacteria and yeasts unlock many of the nutrients in our food that we would otherwise not be able to access, so a combination of both is the way to go for optimum health.

INSOLUBLE FIBRE

This is the indigestible cellulose that forms the cell walls, outer skin and structural parts of plants. It's often called roughage, because it helps push food along the digestive tract and attracts water to keep things moving. When it reaches the colon, gut bacteria can only ferment a small amount. Insoluble fibre is found in grains, nuts, seeds, fruit and vegetables.

SOLUBLE FIBRE

These are the carbs that our gut bugs love. The most soluble and easily fermentable are fructans such as inulin, which are found in many plant foods (everything from wheat to bananas). Then there are beta-glucans (found in oats and barley) and pectins (found in legumes, apples and citrus fruits), which become gooey during digestion, and therefore slow things down. (This is the type of fibre that helps reduce blood glucose and LDL (bad) cholesterol levels.) Psyllium is another type of soluble fibre. It has a strong water-holding capacity but is not easily fermented, which is why it is widely used as a laxative.

RESISTANT STARCH

Resistant starches literally 'resist' being digested in the small intestine and instead pass straight into our colons where they feed the good bacteria that keep us healthy. Resistant starch occurs naturally in all starchy foods, but the best sources are legumes (peas, beans, lentils), whole grains (brown rice, barley, wheat, oats), cashew nuts, seeds and unripe bananas. Our gut bugs love this stuff, and produce loads of butyrate when they ferment it. (Butyrate is the short chain fatty acid that nourishes the gut wall and therefore improves digestion and immune function.)

Another source is starchy foods that have been cooked and then cooled, such as cold potato, pasta and rice. Cooking and cooling changes the structure of the starch, so that it becomes less soluble and slightly more resistant to digestion on its way through. Unfortunately, it's not possible to measure the exact percentage of resistant starch created in this way, as the quantities will vary depending on the type of food, how long it is cooked and cooled.

The gut-brain connection

Scientists have long known that the brain and gut communicate via appetite hormones which, put simply, tell us when we need to eat and when we should stop eating, but they are only just beginning to understand how the health of our microbiome affects this communication.

The walls of our intestines actually contain a network of neurons (the enteric nervous system) which communicate with our brains via the vagus nerve. In fact, 90 per cent of the serotonin in our bodies is made in the gut. (Serotonin is a neurotransmitter which, in the brain, helps regulate mood, appetite, sleep, body temperature, memory and learning. In the gut it is used to control peristaltic contractions that keeps our food and fluids moving. This is partly why people who have anxiety and depression often have digestive issues.)

Studies have found that certain gut bacteria can manufacture special proteins (peptides) that are very similar to hunger-regulating hormones, which means that they may be able to influence eating behaviour. This could be great news for overweight and obese people whose appetite regulating hormones are known to be out of whack.

For me, the most exciting research explores the relationship between our gut health and mental health. For so long I have seen people suffering from mental health issues related to their physical health: from despair and anxiety about their body shape and size to the depression that so often accompanies chronic diseases such as diabetes. Wouldn't it be wonderful if we could positively influence our mood and emotional wellbeing by fuelling our body with less refined carbs and more prebiotic smart carbs? A recent review published in the *British Medical Journal* reports that people with anxiety experienced reduced symptoms when they changed their diet to include more prebiotic smart carbs. Of course, this doesn't prove that happy gut bugs = happy humans (like any nutrition study, there could be many other variables that researchers can't control), but still . . . It's a start.

What is low-carb?

So far I've talked about the main types of carbs and how too many of the crappy ones can negatively impact our health (especially if we are also eating too much fat — the two often go hand in hand. Fried food with sweet sauce anyone?) So yes, we have to reduce our intake of the crap carbs, but exactly what does low-carb mean? How much are we talking?

Unfortunately, there is no widely accepted definition. We do know, however, that a very low carbohydrate diet (20–50 g per day) puts the body into a metabolic state known as ketosis. This is the keto diet you may have heard about, where extreme carb restriction forces the body to metabolise fatty acids to make ketones, which are then used for fuel. (The same thing happens during starvation.)

Researchers have found that a very low carbohydrate ketogenic diet (VLCKD) does lead to weight loss (as long as subjects are carefully monitored and undertake a proper exercise regime), and that it can significantly improve health markers for people with metabolic syndrome, insulin resistance, and type 2 diabetes. However, like any diet that omits a major food group it can be very difficult to meet all known nutrient and fibre targets and it is also very challenging to sustain long term. Plus, activity and movement is a key part of my health and I want it to be for you too. We need adequate amounts of 'smart carbs' to fuel our movement and replenish our muscle glycogen. So, I'm not going to cut out entire food groups or compromise nutrition.

This seems a sensible breakdown of carbohydrate intake. It is based on information on Diabetes Australia's website (the gram amounts are rounded up slightly):

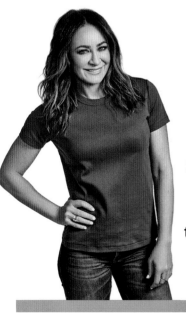

To carb or not to carb is NOT the question, rather it's 'which carbs?' – and the answer is 'smart carbs in the right portions, people!'

Low-carb
= less than 26 per cent of total energy intake (<130 g per day)

Moderate-carb
= between 26 and 45 per cent of total energy intake (130–230 g per day)

High-carb
= more than 45 per cent of total energy intake (>230 g per day)

BUT – and this is important – counting carbs is of no benefit without a consideration of their quality. As I explained earlier, our carbs need to be nutrient-dense and fibre-rich. Put simply, we must choose carbs as they exist in nature. Think veggies like sweet potatoes, broccoli and spinach ... legumes like chickpeas, lentils and kidney beans ... whole grains like oats and quinoa ... salad veggies like avocado, tomato, cucumber and olives and fresh seasonal fruits (especially berries). YUM! Not only do these quality carbs fuel our bodies and brains – they also provide valuable fuel for our gut microbiome, as they are great sources of fibre, resistant starch and prebiotics.

QUALITY CARBS

Whole grains, legumes and veggies are the absolute best options for your health and wellbeing, but like all carbs, some will have higher amounts of easily digestible starches than others. The table below is a rough guide to help you manage your carb intake.

Choosing carbs

Eat in smaller amounts (high in calories) ⟵——⟶ Eat in the largest amounts (low in calories)

Nuts and seeds	Fruit	Milk and milk products	Grains and cereals	Legumes and starchy veggies	Veggies	Low-carb veggies
almonds	apples	hard cheese	oats	beans (kidney,	bean sprouts	alfalfa
brazil nuts	bananas*	kefir	brown rice	lima,	beetroot	sprouts
cashews	berries*	milk	quinoa	cannellini,	bok choy	asparagus
macadamias	citrus fruit	soft cheese	buckwheat	haricot etc)	broccoli	celery
pepitas	stone fruit	yoghurt	millet	chickpeas	brussels	kale
pine nuts			unsweetened	corn	sprouts	lettuce
sesame			cereal	edamame	carrot	radishes
seeds			flakes	fresh peas	cauliflower	rocket
sunflower			unsweetened	legume pasta	cucumber	spinach
seeds			granola	lentils	eggplant	tomatoes
walnuts			wholegrain	parsnips	fennel	watercress
			bread	potato	green beans	
			wholegrain	(skin on)	green	
			pasta	pumpkin	cabbage	
				sweet potato	leek	
				(skin on)	mushrooms	
					onion	
					red cabbage	
					silverbeet	
					zucchini	

* Firm not-quite-ripe bananas are naturally high in resistant starch, and all berries are high in fibre, which reduces the effect on our blood sugar levels.

Balancing carbs with protein and fat

There's not much point taking great care with your carb intake if you are going to load up on saturated fats or eat slabs of steak as big as your head. Here's a *rough guide* to the balance of macronutrients for low, moderate and high carbohydrate intakes. Where possible, always aim for roughly half a plate of plant food for gut health.

A high-carb plate

50%
grains, legumes, starchy veggies*, fruit
*e.g. potatoes, corn, peas

25%
lean meat, fish, egg, dairy, tofu

20%
leafy greens, salad veggies, herbs

5%
healthy fat
(e.g. olive oil, nuts, avocado)

A moderate-carb plate

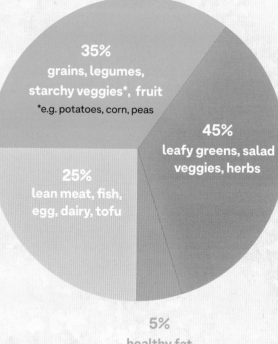

35%
grains, legumes, starchy veggies*, fruit
*e.g. potatoes, corn, peas

45%
leafy greens, salad veggies, herbs

25%
lean meat, fish, egg, dairy, tofu

5%
healthy fat
(e.g. olive oil, nuts, avocado)

The skinny on healthy fats

* Use olive oil for cooking (at a moderate temperature) and for dressing salads.
* Minimise saturated fat (keep your meat lean and any serves of butter, cream, coconut oil or coconut cream to a minimum).
* Eat oily cold-water fish (e.g. sardines) for omega-3.
* Minimise margarine, seed and vegetable oils that are high in omega-6 and have little or no omega-3.
* I recommend skim milk as it has the same amount of calcium and other minerals but fewer calories.

A low-carb plate

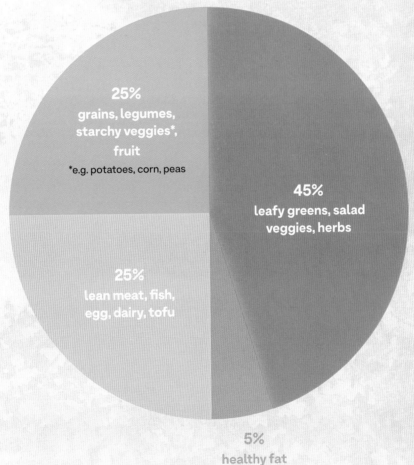

25%
grains, legumes,
starchy veggies*,
fruit
*e.g. potatoes, corn, peas

45%
leafy greens, salad
veggies, herbs

25%
lean meat, fish,
egg, dairy, tofu

5%
healthy fat
(e.g. olive oil, nuts, avocado)

My favourite smart carbs

Smart carbs must have good bang for buck nutritionally.
Check out my top five that hit the spot!

LENTILS
√ low in calories, rich
in iron and folate and
an excellent source
of protein and fibre.

SWEET POTATO
√ high in fibre, vitamin C,
potassium, pantothenic
acid (vitamin B5),
niacin (vitamin B3),
vitamin B6, manganese,
magnesium and copper.
I prefer the orange
ones, as they are high in
beta-carotene, which
is both a pigment and a
potent antioxidant.

COLD COOKED POTATO

√ good source of resistant starch.

CHICKPEAS

√ contain vitamin K, folate, phosphorus, zinc, copper, manganese, choline, selenium and fibre.

FRESH, WHOLE FRUIT

√ contain vitamins, potassium, antioxidants, fibre and folate.

Simple carb swaps

By making a few of these simple changes to your carb intake, you will not only amp the nutrient value of every meal but also the fibre content, which in turn will help with blood glucose control and gut health.

INSTEAD OF WHITE PASTA:

Try pasta made from legumes (chickpeas or lentils) or even quinoa or buckwheat. Better still, try spiralising some carrots and zucchini to make colourful vegetable noodles.

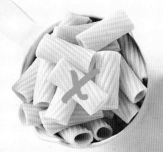

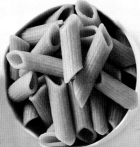

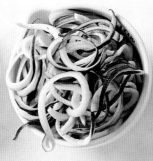

1 cup cooked pasta

45 g 2 g*
Carbs Fibre
*0 g insoluble

1 cup cooked legume-based pasta

34 g 6 g*
Carbs Fibre
*3 g insoluble

1 cup zucchini noodles

6 g 2 g*
Carbs Fibre
*mostly insoluble

Mish Tips

I love transforming a pasta dish from a carb loaded one to a veggie packed one! Check out my Zucchini noodles with lentils and feta on page 103.

INSTEAD OF WHITE RICE:

Grate some cauliflower and sauté in a pan with a few drops of olive oil. Or cook and cool some brown rice or quinoa.

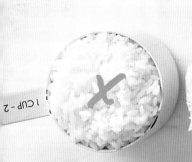

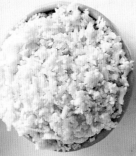

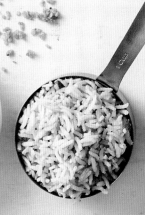

1 cup cooked white rice

46 g 0.6 g*
Carbs Fibre
*none of it insoluble

1 cup grated cauli

5 g 3.5 g
Carbs Fibre

1 cup cooked quinoa

40 g 3 g
Carbs Fibre

1 cup cooked and cooled brown rice

44 g 3.5 g*
Carbs Fibre
*mostly insoluble

INSTEAD OF BOILED POTATO:

Boil a sweet potato. It is loaded with nutrients, most of which are in the skin. Or try boiling a standard potato and cooling it overnight. While the potato cools, it develops resistant starch which is an incredible prebiotic fuel for your happy little gut bugs because it functions like a soluble fibre.

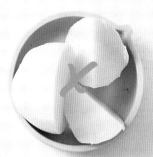
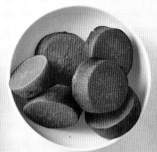
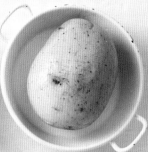

Mish Tips

150 g (1 medium) white potato, peeled, boiled

30 g   2.7 g

Carbs   Fibre

*0 g insoluble

150 g sweet potato, peel on, boiled

25 g   3.5 g

Carbs   Fibre

*mostly insoluble

150 g potato, peel on, boiled and cooled

30 g   2.7 g

Carbs   Fibre

*and some resistant starch

I love sweet potato as an energy booster, it's a great source of fibre and nutrients. Check out my Sweet potato tuna poke bowl recipe on page 170.

INSTEAD OF WHITE BREAD:

Choose bread made from whole grains, preferably sourdough, for easier digestion. If it contains seeds (such as flaxseed, linseed, sunflower, sesame, chia etc), it will have slightly more carbs but the bonus of more fibre.

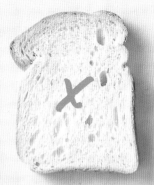
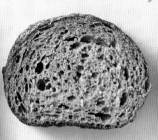
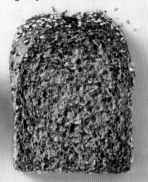

Mish Tips

1 slice white bread

14 g   1 g

Carbs   Fibre

1 slice wholegrain sourdough bread

17 g   2 g

Carbs   Fibre

1 slice wholegrain bread with seeds

18 g   3 g

Carbs   Fibre

I love a slice of toast topped with avocado and feta, or an egg. Adding protein or fat slows down carb absorption even further, giving you sustained energy release and preventing a blood sugar roller-coaster.

My day on a plate

One of the most common questions I am asked is, 'What do you eat?' (as if I don't eat much . . . which I assure you is not the case!). Actually, the right answer is that I practise what I preach — so pick any recipe in this (or any of my books) and it would be a goer for me!

My day-to-day choices will obviously vary, depending on whether I am working out, but on a day that I exercise, this is roughly how it looks:

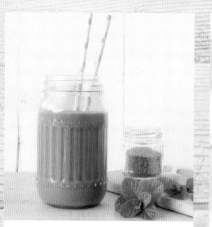

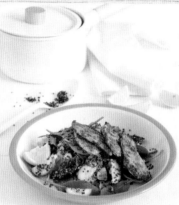

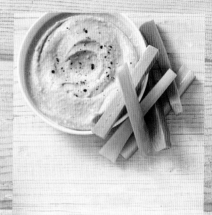

Breakfast

AFTER MY WORKOUT; AROUND 10 AM

Green smoothie:
kale, spinach, apple, celery, avocado, ice and water

Egg on avo toast:
1–2 small pieces of avo
1 x poached egg on 1 slice sourdough with lemon and salt and pepper

Lunch

AROUND 2 PM

Whole food salad:
kale or spinach +
quinoa or sweet potato
or brown rice + shredded barbecue chicken
or tinned sardines +
tomatoes, cucumbers and olive oil

Snack

6–7 macadamia nuts +
2–3 dates

Celery and carrot sticks + hummus

Having a busy home and two boys in the house often means I need to add in a few carb boosters for Steve (and occasionally the Axe Man, too). We do have a few favourite carb boosters in our house, my baked sweet potato wedges being one (see page 221 for a recipe) or a simple scoop of brown rice. A cob of corn always goes down a treat, too.

FASTING AND LOW-CARB EATING

As you can see, I certainly eat well. And I always try to eat only when I am genuinely hungry. In fact, science now tells us it's good for us to feel very hungry at times, as it gives our digestive system a rest break and actually improves our brain function. The easiest way to fast is to ensure there is a 12–16 hour break between your dinner on one day and your breakfast the next (aka no snacks or drinks after dinner).

For me this works well, as I prefer to do my workouts first thing in the morning on an empty stomach. Of course, this doesn't work for everyone, especially if you have a mad rush to get children to school and can't exercise until mid-morning. But if you can manage the occasional hunger pang, a big glass of water or a peppermint tea will tide you over and you will really savour every mouthful of your next meal!

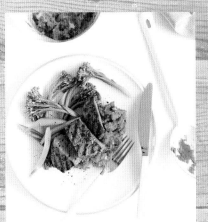

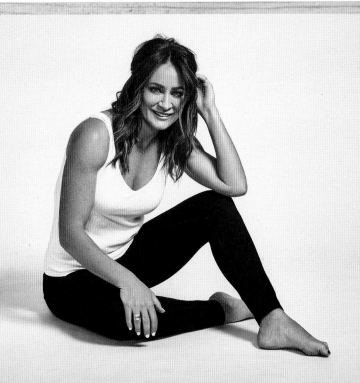

 Dinner

6–7 PM

Grilled meat and veg:
fish or steak + broccoli/
cauliflower mash

or

Grilled meat and veg:
fish or steak +
Greek salad

 Eating out

On occasion I eat out and thoroughly enjoy the bread and butter and a glass of wine (or two!) and share a dessert. And, yes, I sometimes have some dark chocolate or licorice at home. It's all about balance.

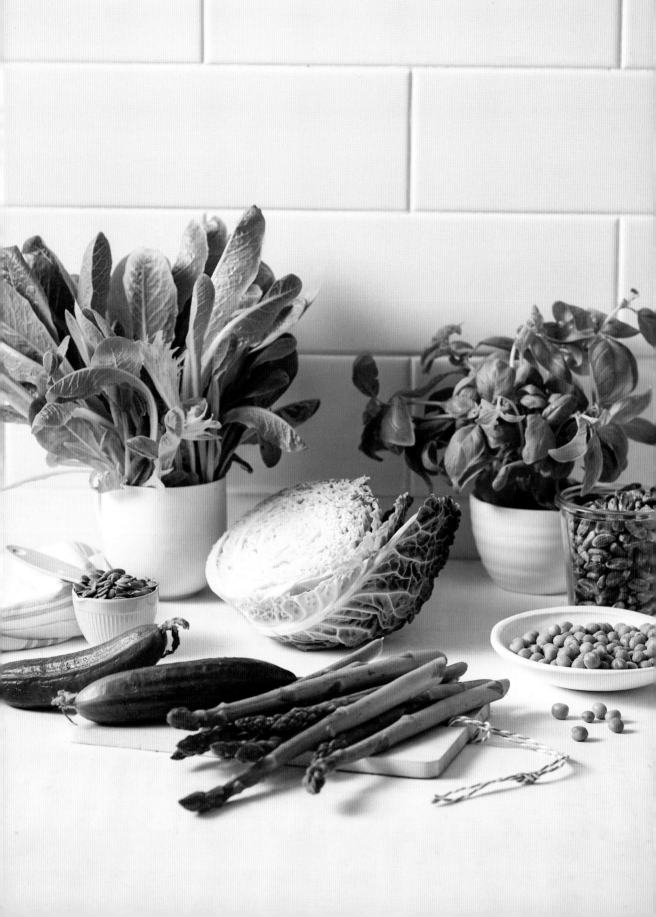

Case study

Nerida's story

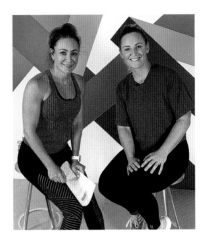

Nerida is one of my 12WBT stars. She started the program in 2011 with the goal of losing 20 kilos. She was initially quite fearful about exercising, but soon fell so in love with it that she switched careers and is now in the fitness industry herself!

Nerida says that understanding how her food choices affected her body was key:

'Nutrition plays such a big part of maintaining a healthy weight – [it] didn't matter how much I trained, if I wasn't eating nutritious food and fuelling my body correctly, I wouldn't feel good and be at my best.'

She also learned that the right carbs are important:

'Carbs are necessary for performance. Any diet that cuts out a whole food group is not sustainable. Sure, some diets that cut out certain foods provide results, but they can [also] leave you feeling deflated and lethargic. Carbs are necessary as they fuel and give us the energy to be active and work out – working out [is] an integral part of my life and provide[s] me with mental clarity and increases [my] overall happiness.'

Nerida says that the most valuable lesson she learned was about her relationship with food:

'12WBT really taught me about emotional eating. I had no idea that I was an emotional eater until I watched the videos on 12WBT. I didn't understand that I was hiding my emotions through binge eating – I didn't even know it was a thing! This was a huge shift for me. The tools and strategies on how to change my relationship between my emotions and food was one of the most valuable lessons I got from 12WBT.'

The benefits of her lifestyle changes?

'The benefits I have gotten from changing my habits have been everlasting and have stuck with me to this day. I now have sustained energy levels, [I] maintain a healthy weight, have no brain fog, I sleep better, I have better self-esteem and I enjoy food in social situations.'

The exercise bit

So far I've talked about how choosing the right carbs can improve your metabolism, energy levels and mood, but do not think for one moment that I have forgotten about movement!

I have always said that to live your best life you need to care about what you put into your body and what you do with your body. Now you might think that exercise is important for the physiological side of our wellbeing – keeping our heart healthy, our bones strong and our weight under control. But more research is showing that movement is crucial not only for our mental health but also our cognitive function – a body that moves gives you a brain that grooves.

It's so easy to feel maxed out in today's super busy world. Most of us are juggling so many balls in the air that the idea of adding exercise to our day seems too much. We're trying to reduce our stress, not add to it, right? But I promise you, even just a quick hit of 10 minutes will boost blood supply to your brain, helping you to think faster on your feet, and boost your mood. Exercise doesn't need to be a big deal – it can simply be part of how you get around each day. In the table below I've listed a bunch of options that start from super short 'incidental' exercises through to more 'formal' options. I've also put together a few circuits you can do in the backyard, the lounge room or wherever works for you.

Choosing exercise

	Incidental	Formal
CARDIO	* Hop off your bus or train 1 or 2 stops early and walk the difference. * Do high knee runs down the hallway. * Put on some tunes and dance.	* Bike ride with sprints and hills. * Cardio class (e.g. BodyAttack, Cycle). * Hurdles. * Cardio workout (see opposite page).
STRENGTH	* Wall sit while you brush your teeth. * Do push ups before you watch a TV show. * Do rolling bridges after you watch a TV show or during the ad break.	* Strength workout (see page 34).
CARDIO + STRENGTH	* Run up and down the steps or stairs. * Do jump squats while you're waiting for the jug to boil. * Piggyback your kids up a hill.	* Gymnastics. * HIIT class (e.g. Grit, BodyStep). * Tough Mudder or Spartan Race. * Cardio + strength workout (see page 35).

Cardio workout

AMRAP (as many rounds as possible in the time you have)

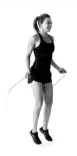

1 | 1 min
skipping

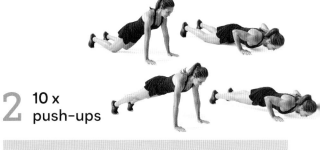

2 | 10 x
push-ups

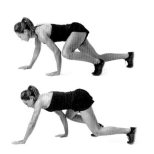

3 | 1 min
bear crawls

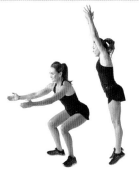

4 | 10 x
squat jumps

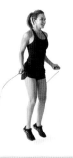

5 | 1 min
skipping

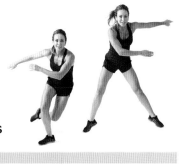

6 | 10 x
ice skaters

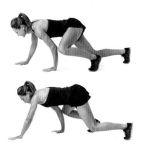

7 | 1 min
bear crawls

Eating more carbs than
we need, day after day,
and doing very little
exercise is a one-way
street to weight gain
and disease.

Strength workout

21:15:9 (reps) in AMRAP (as many rounds as possible in the time you have)

ROUND ONE

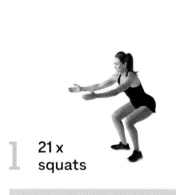

1 **21 x squats**

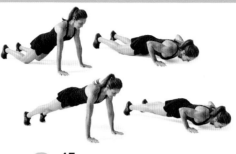

2 **15 x push-ups**

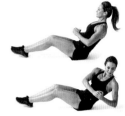

3 **9 x Russian twists**

(L + R = 1 rep)

ROUND TWO

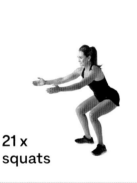

1 **21 x squats**

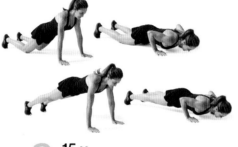

2 **15 x push-ups**

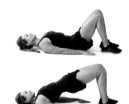

3 **9 x rolling bridges**

ROUND THREE

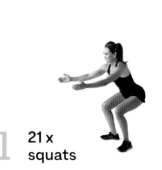

1 **21 x squats**

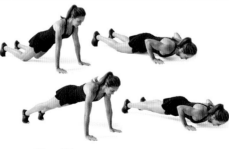

2 **15 x push-ups**

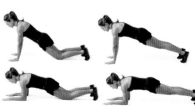

3 **9 x hand to forearm planks**

Start on hands, drop to R forearm, drop to L forearm, lift to R hand, lift to L hand = 1 rep

Cardio + strength workout

Do 1 or 2 rounds of this combined cardio and strength workout

1   **1 min**
skipping
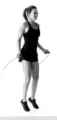

2   **1 min**
bear crawls
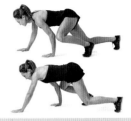

3   **1 min**
triceps dips
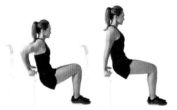

4   **1 min**
Russian twists
(L + R = 1 rep)
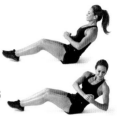

5   **1 min**
squat jumps
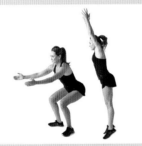

6   **1 min**
hand to forearm planks
Start on hands, drop to R forearm, drop to L forearm, lift to R hand, lift to L hand = 1 rep
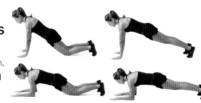

7   **1 min**
rolling bridges
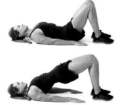

8   **1 min**
push-ups
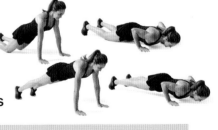

9   **1 min**
ice skaters
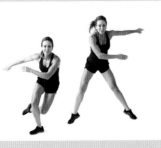

10   **1 min**
skipping
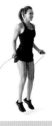

Snacks and exercise

A well-timed snack can be a game changer when training. Effective recovery and replenishment can be achieved with the right choices. Snack 'smart' not 'silly' and you'll be set up for success!

Snacking for the sake of snacking is a super quick way to stack on unwanted kilos. I call this 'Silly Snacking'. Snacking sensibly to recover from the effects of exercise is the other end of the scale, and I call it 'Smart Snacking'. Get smart about carbs by matching your post-workout snack with the type of exercise you've been doing. For example, if you've been doing cardio training (running, jumping, cycling,

swimming, hiking) you should have a carb-based snack to help replenish your muscle glycogen. If you've been doing strength training (lifting, pushing, pulling) you'll want to reach for a protein-based snack to help with muscle repair and restoration. Smart snacking reduces muscle fatigue and tiredness, so you are ready to roll with your life rather than feeling like you just wanna roll into bed!

Suggested snack for exercise type

Exercise type	Suggested snack	Carb value
Cardio (e.g. running)	1 small banana (78 g)	24 g
Cardio/strength 1 (e.g. hiking uphill)	1 red apple (150 g) with nut butter (10 g)	20 g
Strength (e.g. weights)	Natural yoghurt (200 g)	12 g
Cardio/strength 2 (e.g. indoor cycling)	1 slice wholemeal toast (14 g) with avocado (50 g)	18.5 g

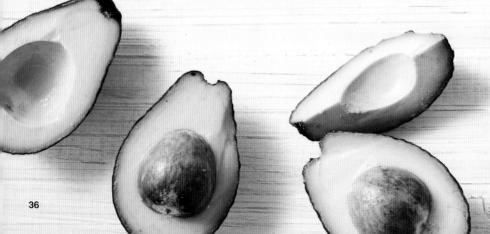

Coping with cravings

You know by now that I'll always be straight up with you, and swapping from a high carb to a reduced carb approach might be pretty challenging at first. If you are accustomed to having sweet things as a high-carb eater, it is likely you will initially still want sweet things as a reduced-carb eater. You've been feeding a sweet tooth and it now has a heightened sense of 'sweet' taste.

You also have to try to separate whether you are craving carbohydrates because your body needs them (particularly after exercise) or if it is just a habit. If it's a habit, then start breaking it by swapping those carb-laden choices for low-carb ones (combined with either some protein or good fats to keep you full). A handful of nuts often hits the spot for me! Or you could try having a teaspoon of fermented veg with your meals. Many people say that building a taste for sour foods helps to balance cravings for sweet ones.

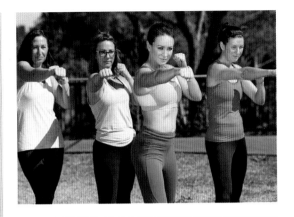

Cravings are like waves, they come and they go – so ride the wave of the crave and back yourself to ride it out. Hang ten, baby!

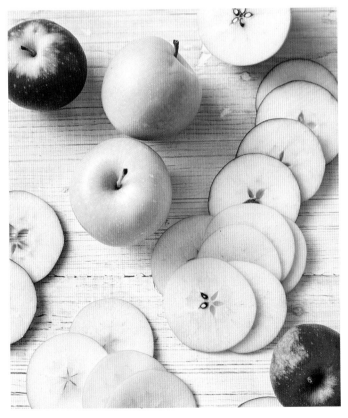

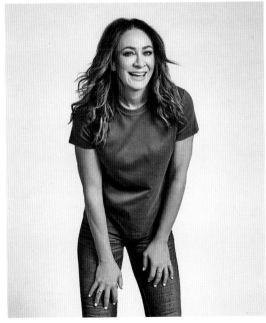

Savoury snacks

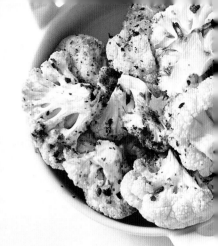

When you're craving something savoury, and it's a while between meals, these savoury snacks are just the 'tide me over' ticket. They're packed with nom nom flavour and nutrition – enjoy!

Crunchy spiced chickpeas

Serves: **1**
Prep time: **5 minutes**
Cooking time: **40 minutes**

100 g drained and rinsed tinned
   chickpeas
olive oil spray
generous pinch of smoked paprika

1. Preheat the oven to 230°C (210°C fan-forced). Line a baking tray with baking paper.
2. Pat the chickpeas dry with paper towel, then spread out on the prepared tray and lightly spray with olive oil. Sprinkle the paprika over the chickpeas and toss to coat evenly.
3. Spread the chickpeas out again and bake for 30–40 minutes or until lightly browned and dry to touch. Remove from the oven – they will crunch up as they cool.

Garlic and thyme grilled mushrooms

Serves: **2**
Prep time: **10 minutes**
Cooking time: **10 minutes**

2 field mushrooms, stems removed and
   finely chopped
olive oil spray
1 clove garlic, finely chopped
2 teaspoons lemon thyme leaves
5 g walnuts, chopped
20 g baby spinach leaves

1. Preheat the grill to high.
2. Place the mushrooms, stem side down, on a baking tray and grill for 1–2 minutes.
3. Meanwhile, combine the chopped mushroom stem, garlic, lemon thyme and walnuts in a small bowl and season with freshly ground black pepper.
4. Carefully turn the mushrooms over and lightly spray with olive oil. Sprinkle the filling into the mushroom cups and grill for 5–6 minutes or until golden and the mushrooms are just tender. Serve with the baby spinach leaves.

Prawn parcels

Serves: **2**
Prep time: **20 minutes,**
   plus cooling time
Cooking time: **5 minutes**

1 tablespoon fish sauce
3 teaspoons brown sugar
1 kaffir lime leaf
1 tablespoon lime juice
200 g cooked, peeled and deveined
   king prawns, finely chopped
1 spring onion, finely chopped
2 tablespoons chopped coriander
2 tablespoons chopped mint
6 iceberg lettuce leaves, trimmed

1. Combine the fish sauce, sugar, kaffir lime leaf, lime juice and 1 tablespoon water in a small saucepan and stir over low heat until the sugar has dissolved. Increase the heat and bring to the boil, then reduce the heat and simmer for 1 minute. Remove and set aside to cool. Remove the kaffir lime leaf.
2. Combine the prawn, spring onion, coriander and mint in a bowl. Pour the fish sauce mixture over the top and stir to combine.
3. Spoon the prawn mixture into the lettuce leaves, then fold in the sides and roll into parcels and serve.

116	14.7 g
Calories	Carbs

46	5 g
Calories	Carbs

136	4.9 g
Calories	Carbs

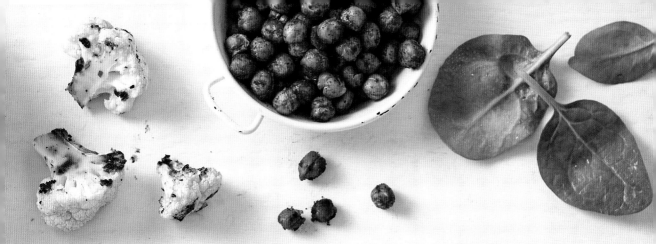

Miso cauliflower bites

Serves: **1**
Prep time: **5 minutes**
Cooking time: **20 minutes**

400 g cauliflower, trimmed and cut
    into florets
olive oil spray
1 x 6 g sachet instant miso soup powder

1. Preheat the oven to 180°C (160°C
fan-forced). Line a baking tray with
baking paper.
2. Place the cauliflower in a large bowl.
Give it a good spray with olive oil and
then sprinkle the miso powder over the
top and toss well to combine.
3. Spread the cauliflower florets over
the prepared tray and bake for 15–20
minutes or until tender and golden,
depending on how crispy you like them.
Serve warm.

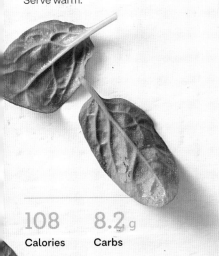

108   8.2 g
Calories   Carbs

Baba ganoush

Serves: **8**
Prep time: **15 minutes**
Cooking time: **35 minutes**

2 eggplants
2 cloves garlic, crushed
1 tablespoon lemon juice
2 tablespoons tahini
3 tablespoons finely chopped flat-leaf
    parsley
pinch of ground cumin

1. Preheat the oven to 200°C (180°C
fan-forced). Preheat a barbecue grill
to high or heat a chargrill pan over
high heat. Place the eggplants directly
on the chargrill and cook, turning
occasionally, for 10–15 minutes or until
the skin is black and blistered.
2. Transfer the eggplants to a baking
tray, place in the oven and roast for 20
minutes or until the flesh is very soft.
Remove and set aside to cool.
3. Scoop the flesh from the eggplants
and discard the skin. Place the flesh
in a food processor, add the garlic and
lemon juice and process until thick and
creamy. Add the tahini and process
until smooth. Stir in the parsley, season
with freshly ground black pepper and
sprinkle with the cumin to serve.

55   2.6 g
Calories   Carbs

Chilli and lime sweet potato chips

Serves: **6**
Prep time: **20 minutes**
Cooking time: **40 minutes**

2 cage-free egg whites, lightly beaten
2 tablespoons finely grated lime zest
½ teaspoon chilli powder or to taste
1 kg sweet potatoes, cut into 1 cm thick
    chips

1. Preheat the oven to 200°C (180°C
fan-forced). Line two large baking trays
with baking paper.
2. Combine the egg white, lime zest
and chilli powder in a large bowl. Add
the sweet potato chips and toss until
well coated. Divide the chips between
the prepared trays, spacing them out
evenly.
3. Bake, turning once, for 35–40 minutes
or until crisp and golden. Serve hot.

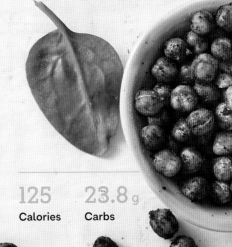

125   23.8 g
Calories   Carbs

Speedy snacks

When time is of the essence, and you need something to just 'grab and go', these are my go-to solutions! They're easy to throw together and they hit the spot till an actual meal time.

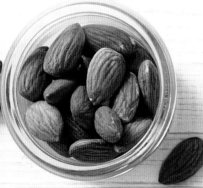

Almonds

Serves: **1**

25 g natural almonds

149 Calories **12** g Carbs

Veggie sticks with hummus

Serves: **1**

1 carrot, cut into batons

3 celery stalks, cut into batons

2 tablespoons hummus

Dip the veggie batons into the hummus.

133 Calories **8.2** g Carbs

Mini tomato, bocconcini and basil skewers

Serves: **4**

4 cherry or small roma tomatoes, halved

4 baby bocconcini, halved

16 basil leaves

Thread the tomato, boccocini and basil onto eight toothpicks and serve.

15 Calories **0.3** g Carbs

Capsicum and cottage cheese

Serves: **1**

1 red capsicum, seeded and cut into batons

⅓ cup low-fat cottage cheese

Dip the capsicum batons into the cottage cheese.

119 Calories **4.7** g Carbs

Egg-power!

Serves: **1**

1 cage-free egg

Boil the egg to your
liking. Allow to cool,
then peel, cut in half
and season with freshly
ground black pepper.

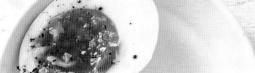

70
Calories

0.2 g
Carbs

Yoghurt

Serves: **1**

1 x 200 g tub low-fat
natural yoghurt

114
Calories

12 g
Carbs

Tinned tuna

Serves: **1**

1 x 95 g tin tuna in spring
water, drained

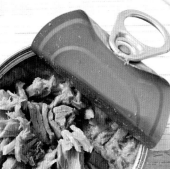

82
Calories

0 g
Carbs

Strawberry ballerinas

Serves: **1**

6 large strawberries,
hulled
60 g fresh low-fat
ricotta

Cut the strawberries
in two, about one-third
of the way down.
Spoon the ricotta onto
the strawberry bases,
put the tops back on
and serve.

109
Calories

5.9 g
Carbs

Capsicum and hummus

Serves: **1**

1 red capsicum,
seeded and cut into
batons
2 tablespoons hummus

Dip the capsicum batons
into the hummus.

124
Calories

7.1 g
Carbs

Sweet snacks

Sometimes you just need a sweet sumthin' sumthin'! These recipes will keep you on the low-carb path, while still delivering the sweet treat that your tastebuds are asking for.

Balsamic and basil strawberries with ricotta

Serves: **2**
Prep time: **10 minutes, plus 30 minutes standing time**

250 g strawberries, washed, hulled and quartered
1 tablespoon caster sugar
1½ teaspoons balsamic vinegar
4 basil leaves
60 g fresh low-fat ricotta

1. Place the strawberries in a glass or ceramic bowl. Add the sugar and balsamic vinegar and toss to coat. Set aside to macerate for 30 minutes.
2. Shred two of the basil leaves and stir through the strawberries, then spoon into serving glasses. Top with a dollop of ricotta and serve with the remaining whole basil leaves.

Sweet spiced yoghurt dip with strawberries

Serves: **2**
Prep time: **5 minutes**

200 g low-fat natural yoghurt
1 teaspoon honey
½ teaspoon ground or freshly grated nutmeg
½ teaspoon ground allspice
¼ teaspoon ground ginger
¼ teaspoon ground cinnamon
250 g strawberries, washed and hulled

1. Combine the yoghurt, honey and spices in a bowl. Serve with the strawberries for dipping.

Mish Tips

Any seasonal fruit will work wonderfully in this dish — try sliced banana, pear, melon, kiwi fruit or berries.

Cacao fudge bites

Makes: **21**
Prep time: **10 minutes, plus 30 minutes setting time**

1 cup walnuts
235 g medjool dates, seeded
½ cup raw cacao powder

1. Place the walnuts, dates and cacao powder in a food processor and blend until finely ground. The mixture should resemble cake crumbs but will stick together easily when pressed.
2. Firmly press the mixture into 21 ice-cube holes and place in the fridge to set for 30 minutes. Eat straight from the fridge.

Mish Tips

These are magic but at 80 calories each, make sure that you only take one of them out of the fridge! If you are one of those people who can't stop at one, the answer is easy: don't make these!

104	14 g
Calories	Carbs

102	13.5 g
Calories	Carbs

80	9.1 g
Calories	Carbs

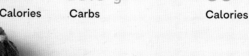

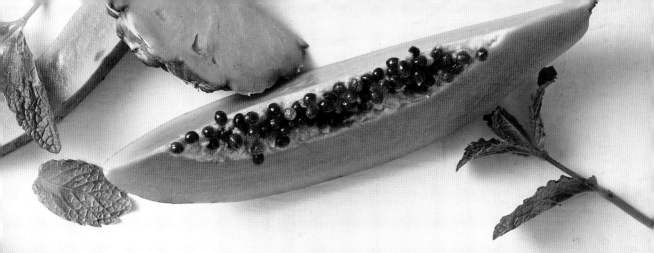

Snack balls

Makes: **30**

Prep time: **20 minutes**

1 cup raw cashews
1 cup natural almonds
1 cup sunflower seeds
2 cups dried dates
1 cup dried currants
1 teaspoon vanilla essence
½ cup desiccated coconut

1. Place the nuts and seeds in a large food processor and blitz until finely chopped. Add the dates, currants and vanilla essence and process until almost smooth and quite sticky.
2. Tip the coconut into a shallow bowl.
3. Using wet hands, roll the mixture into 30 walnut-sized balls (or 60 smaller balls if preferred) and toss to coat in the coconut. Place in an airtight container between layers of baking paper to stop them sticking together. Store in the fridge for up to a month.

142 **Calories**   11.7 g **Carbs**

Papaya with lime and coconut cream

Serves: **2**

Prep time: **5 minutes**

1 papaya or paw paw, seeded and cut into wedges
finely grated zest and juice of 1 lime
3 tablespoons low-fat coconut cream
1 teaspoon brown sugar

1. Divide the papaya between serving dishes. Drizzle with the lime juice and spoon over the coconut cream.
2. Sprinkle with the sugar and lime zest and serve.

Mish Tips

Look for rosy-hued red papaya at your local green grocer or in the fruit and veg section of your supermarket. It's much sweeter and more aromatic than its yellow-fleshed counterpart, paw paw, though they both work well here.

110 **Calories**   13.7 g **Carbs**

Pineapple carpaccio with ginger and mint yoghurt

Serves: **2**

Prep time: **10 minutes**

80 g low-fat natural yoghurt
2 tablespoons finely chopped mint, plus extra leaves to serve
2 teaspoons finely chopped glace ginger
10 thin slices pineapple

1. Combine the yoghurt, chopped mint and ginger in a bowl.
2. Arrange the pineapple slices in a single layer, overlapping slightly, on a serving plate. Top with the yoghurt mixture and serve with the extra mint leaves.

Mish Tips

If ginger isn't your thing, simply leave it out or replace it with a pinch of brown sugar or a little finely grated orange zest.

75 **Calories**   13.4 g **Carbs**

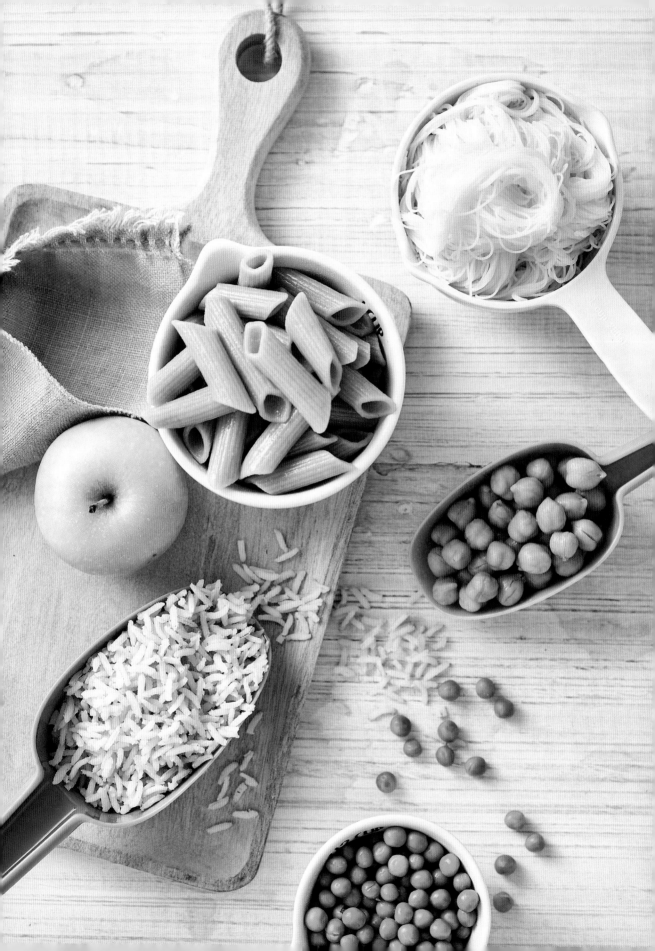

Four low-carb meal plans

The next few pages should be your go-to as you start to transition to a low and smart carb way of eating.

We have created four amazing meal plans to take all the guesswork out and put all the flavour in. You will get some of my great tips, learn new tricks and end up with a nutritious home-cooked meal that everyone can enjoy. Psst . . . for those of you that like to get a little creative, we have also included a blank plan so you can create your own masterpiece!

CARB BOOSTERS

As I said a little earlier, a one-size-fits-all approach does not work with low-carb eating. Some of you may be feeding a household of teenage boys, some of you may be feeding an elderly parent and everything else that a modern family is made up of. Do not fret, as I have you covered with my really simple and very tasty carb booster options.

Carb boosters to enjoy

Food	Weight	Carb Content
1 banana	120 g	24 g
½ cup cooked/canned chickpeas	100 g	21 g
1 slice wholemeal bread	30 g	13 g
1 cup cooked pasta	180 g	48 g
½ cup cooked peas	80 g	11 g
1 large baked potato	150 g	30 g
6 prunes	60 g	33 g
1 Ryvita	25 g	16 g
1 corn cob	150 g	28 g
1 cup cooked rice vermicelli noodles	180 g	45 g
1 cup cooked couscous	150 g	35 g
1 cup cooked brown rice	150 g	33 g
1 apple	120 g	16 g
1 cup oven-baked sweet potato chips	150 g	25g

Easy ingredient swaps

We all have different tastes, so match alternatives for texture, nutrients and flavour to ensure that every recipe is a winner in your household.

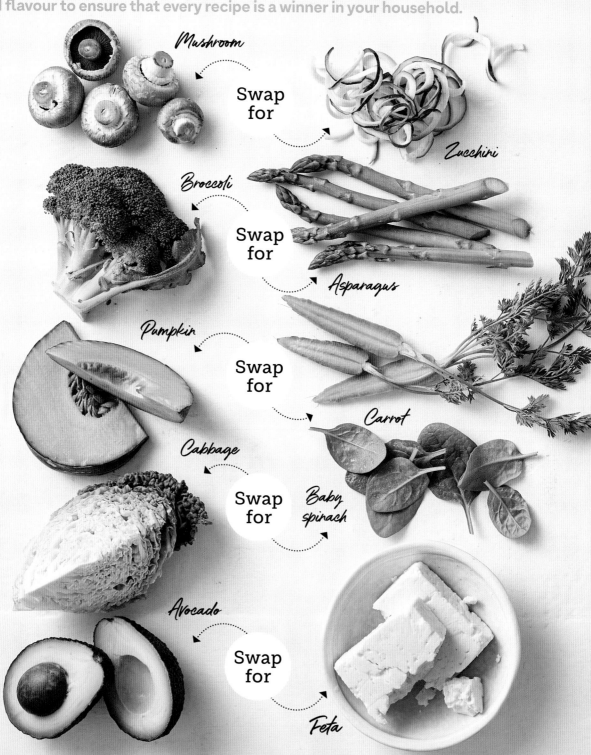

Mushroom

Swap for

Zucchini

Broccoli

Swap for

Asparagus

Pumpkin

Swap for

Carrot

Cabbage

Swap for

Baby spinach

Avocado

Swap for

Feta

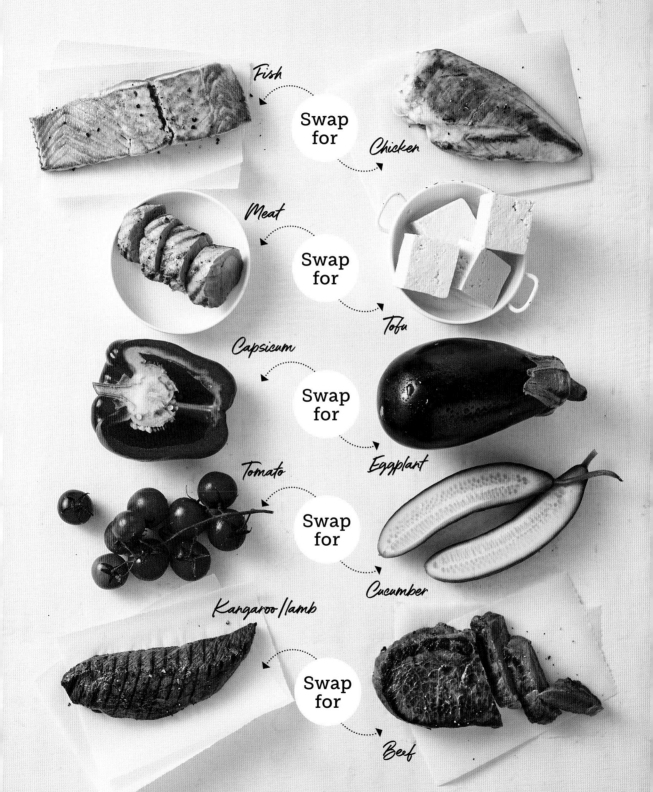

Fish

Swap for

Chicken

Meat

Swap for

Tofu

Capsicum

Swap for

Eggplant

Tomato

Swap for

Cucumber

Kangaroo / lamb

Swap for

Beef

Weekly Plan: Week 1

Enjoy two well-positioned snacks each day (see pages 38–43 for ideas). If you're not a snacker, add a Carb Booster to your meals (see page 45). Remember you will still need to be under 130 grams of carbs per day to be eating 'low carb'.

	Meatless Monday	Tuesday	Wednesday
Breakfast	Super green smoothie (page 213)	Italian-style baked eggs (page 85)	Super green smoothie (page 213)
Lunch	Rainbow salad jar (page 172)	LEFTOVER Braised pumpkin and lentils with haloumi	LEFTOVER Chicken curry patties with veggie noodles
Dinner	Braised pumpkin and lentils with haloumi (page 168)	Chicken curry patties with veggie noodles (page 64)	Veal goulash (page 179)
TOTAL CARBS	83.7 g	40.6 g	60.1 g

Thursday	Friday	Saturday	Sunday
Italian-style baked eggs (page 85)	Super green smoothie (page 213)	Souffle omelette with spinach and mushrooms (page 99)	Grated beetroot and chickpea fritters (page 104)
LEFTOVER Veal goulash	**LEFTOVER** Quick prawn curry	**FREEZABLE COOK-UP** Sweet potato and cannellini bean soup (page 229)	Chicken and lettuce 'tacos' (page 116)
Quick prawn curry (page 89)	Steak with creamy mushroom sauce (page 92)	Fish kebabs with green leaf salad (page 78)	Roast lamb with lemon, garlic and rosemary (page 140)
33.1 g	**43.8** g	**44.1** g	**53.8** g

Weekly Plan: Week 2

Enjoy two well-positioned snacks each day (see pages 38–43 for ideas). If you're not a snacker, add a Carb Booster to your meals (see page 45). Remember you will still need to be under 130 grams of carbs per day to be eating 'low carb'.

	Meatless Monday	Tuesday	Wednesday
Breakfast	Summer smoothie bowl (page 214)	Scrambled eggs with spinach and avocado (page 95)	Summer smoothie bowl (page 214)
Lunch	**FROM THE FREEZER** Sweet potato and cannellini bean soup (page 229)	**LEFTOVER** Zucchini noodles with lentils and feta	**LEFTOVER** Kangaroo with mint yoghurt and pea salad
Dinner	Zucchini noodles with lentils and feta (page 103)	Kangaroo with mint yoghurt and pea salad (page 132)	Sweet potato and tuna poke bowl (page 170)
TOTAL CARBS	82.2 g	34.3 g	72.2 g

Thursday	Friday	Saturday	Sunday
Scrambled eggs with spinach and avocado (page 95)	Super green smoothie (page 213)	Baked mushrooms (page 120)	Lentil salad with poached eggs (page 114)
LEFTOVER Sweet potato and tuna poke bowl	**LEFTOVER** Spicy chicken and broccoli stir-fry	**FREEZABLE COOK-UP** Hearty lentil soup (page 246)	Lamb steaks with spiced sweet potato and coriander mash (page 184)
Spicy chicken and broccoli stir-fry (page 145)	Mexican-style cottage pie (page 181)	Seared salmon with vegetable noodles (page 90)	Ginger and lemongrass roast chicken (page 110)
43.8 g	**68.5** g	**55.6** g	**54.6** g

Weekly Plan: Week 3

Enjoy two well-positioned snacks each day (see pages 38–43 for ideas). If you're not a snacker, add a Carb Booster to your meals (see page 45). Remember you will still need to be under 130 grams of carbs per day to be eating 'low carb'.

	Meatless Monday	Tuesday	Wednesday
Breakfast	Super green smoothie (page 213)	Italian-style baked eggs (page 85)	Super green smoothie (page 213)
Lunch	FROM THE FREEZER Hearty lentil soup (page 246)	LEFTOVER Chickpea korma curry	LEFTOVER Pork with sweet potato chips and broccoli salad
Dinner	Chickpea korma curry (page 240)	Pork with sweet potato chips and broccoli salad (page 202)	Lamb with Moroccan carrot salad (page 156)
TOTAL CARBS	98.9 g	64.9 g	73.9 g

Thursday	Friday	Saturday	Sunday
Italian-style baked eggs (page 85)	Super green smoothie (page 213)	Scrambled eggs with spinach and avocado (page 95)	Roasted vegetable frittata (page 191)
LEFTOVER Lamb with Moroccan carrot salad	**LEFTOVER** Grilled fish with herbed veggie 'couscous'	**FREEZABLE COOK-UP** Celeriac and white bean soup (page 176)	Charred chicken, corn and mango salad (page 194)
Grilled fish with herbed veggie 'couscous' (page 74)	Beef and mushrooms with mash (page 123)	Low-FODMAP pumpkin and spinach lasagne (page 144)	Hoisin beef stir-fry with spring vegetables (page 150)
30.5 g	**52.3** g	**42.6** g	**58.8** g

Weekly Plan: Week 4

Enjoy two well-positioned snacks each day (see pages 38–43 for ideas). If you're not a snacker, add a Carb Booster to your meals (see page 45). Remember you will still need to be under 130 grams of carbs per day to be eating 'low carb'.

	Meatless Monday	Tuesday	Wednesday
Breakfast	Summer smoothie bowl (page 214)	Scrambled eggs with spinach and avocado (page 95)	Summer smoothie bowl (page 214)
Lunch	FROM THE FREEZER Celeriac and white bean soup (page 176)	LEFTOVER Eggplant, sweet potato and ricotta bake	LEFTOVER Lamb with beetroot puree and herbed peas
Dinner	Eggplant, sweet potato and ricotta bake (page 173)	Lamb with beetroot puree and herbed peas (page 149)	Miso salmon with cauliflower fried rice (page 66)
TOTAL CARBS	79.5 g	41.3 g	52 g

Thursday	Friday	Saturday	Sunday
Scrambled eggs with spinach and avocado (page 95)	Super green smoothie (page 213)	Japanese tofu and cabbage pancake (page 88)	Mushroom omelettes with spinach and cherry tomatoes (page 81)
LEFTOVER Miso salmon with cauliflower fried rice	**LEFTOVER** Chicken and vegetables in coconut	**FREEZABLE COOK-UP** Beef and bean soup (page 208)	Chicken kebabs with radish and cucumber salad (page 80)
Chicken and vegetables in coconut (page 154)	Saganaki-style prawns (page 162)	Dukkah-crusted pork with roasted vegetable salad (page 183)	Roast beef dinner (page 180)
24.1 g	**61.8** g	**50.2** g	**32.7** g

Weekly Plan: My Week

Use the recipes in this book to create your own Weekly Plan below. Remember to tally your total carbs so you are consuming under 130 grams per day. Don't forget to count your snacks!

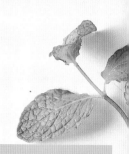

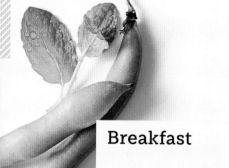

	Meatless Monday	Tuesday	Wednesday
Breakfast			
Lunch			
Dinner			
TOTAL CARBS			

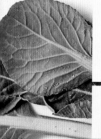

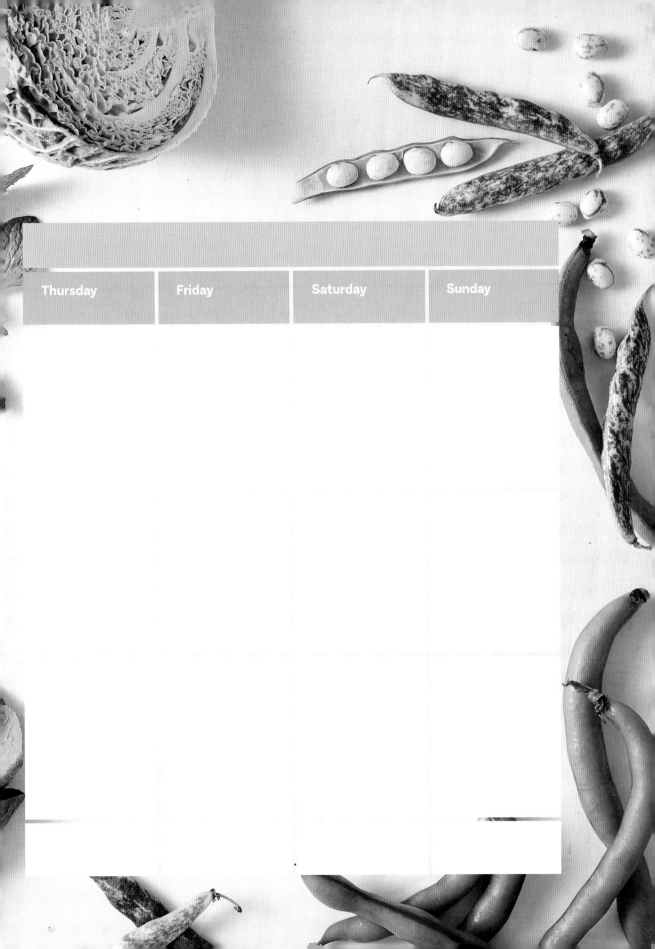

Thursday	Friday	Saturday	Sunday

PART TWO

The recipes

Navigating the recipes

In the following pages you'll find my all-time favourite low-carb recipes — easy, no-fuss and practical. The recipes are broken down into carb content for simple navigation:

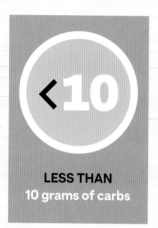

LESS THAN
10 grams of carbs

LESS THAN
20 grams of carbs

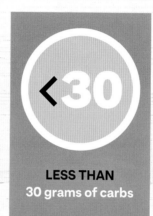

LESS THAN
30 grams of carbs

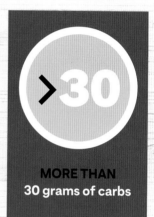

MORE THAN
30 grams of carbs

Nutritional information

Each recipe includes nutritional information in the left-hand panel for easy reference. Use this to ensure you're consuming less than 130 grams of carbs a day.

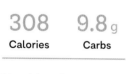

308	9.8 g
Calories	Carbs

Nutritional Information
(per serve)

Calories	**308**
Protein	**26.5 g**
Fat Total	**16.9 g**
Fat Saturated	**4.2 g**
Carbohydrates	**9.8 g**
Sugars	**7.1 g**
Sodium	**789.0 mg**
Dietary Fibre	**6.6 g**

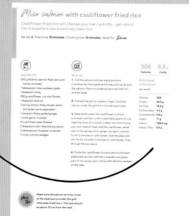
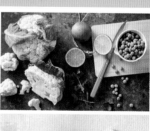
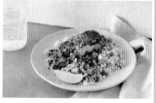

How to use up leftovers

Tightly wrap leftover vegetables, such as onion, leek, capsicum, sweet potato and pumpkin, in plastic film and keep in the fridge for up to 3 days.

Alternatively, steam or boil chopped sweet potato or pumpkin, then cool and place in airtight bags or containers in useable portions. Freeze for up to 3 months.

Wrap leftover leafy herbs, such as coriander, in damp paper towel and place in a sealed plastic bag. Keep in the fridge for up to 1 week.

Wrap leftover sage in damp paper towel and place in a sealed plastic bag. Keep in the fridge for up to 4 days.

Place leftover tinned lentils, beans or chickpeas in a zip-lock bag, expel the air and seal tightly, then store in the freezer for up to 1 month. Alternatively, store them in an airtight container in the fridge for up to 1 week.

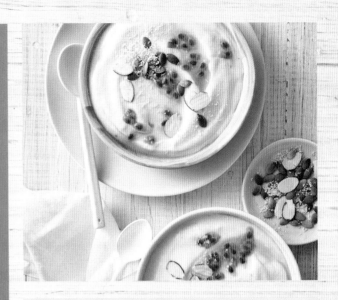

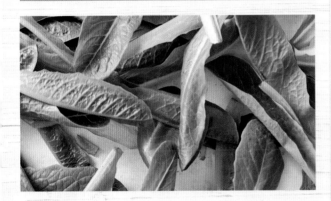

Great for . . .

I've included a 'Great for' feature in each recipe, and, yep, you guessed it, this indicates which meal a recipe would be good for. Most recipes are perfect for Lunch, Dinner or Leftovers, but the Breakfasts are a little harder to find. Use the Breakfast recipe index in the next column for quick reference.

Quick breakfast recipe index

Asian chicken omelette	73
Baked mushrooms	120
Grated beetroot and chickpea fritters	104
Italian-style baked eggs	85
Japanese tofu and cabbage pancake	88
Lentil salad with poached eggs	114
Mushroom omelettes with spinach and cherry tomatoes	81
Potato, spinach and feta tortilla	152
Roasted capsicum and ham frittata with avocado and herb salad	77
Roasted vegetable frittata	191
Scrambled eggs with spinach and avocado	95
Souffle omelette with spinach and mushrooms	99
Summer smoothie bowl	214
Super green smoothie	213
Tropical fruit salad with toasted coconut yoghurt	216
Zucchini cakes with dill raita	158

< LESS THAN

10

grams of carbs

Chicken curry patties with veggie noodles

Winner winner chicken dinner! This is one of Axel's favourites, and mine too. Make a double batch of the patties and freeze half (uncooked) for a quick meal another time.

Serves: **2** • Prep time: **15 minutes** • Cooking time: **10 minutes** • Great for: *Lunch or Leftovers*

Ingredients

300 g lean chicken mince
2 teaspoons yellow curry paste
1 tablespoon finely chopped coriander, plus extra leaves to serve
olive oil spray
1 clove garlic, crushed
2 teaspoons grated ginger
250 g carrot, cut into noodles
250 g zucchini, cut into noodles

Method

1. Combine the mince, curry paste and chopped coriander in a bowl and season well with freshly ground black pepper. Shape the mixture into six even patties.

2. Lightly spray a large non-stick frying pan with olive oil and heat over medium heat. Add the patties and cook for 3 minutes each side or until golden and cooked through. Remove and keep warm.

3. Lightly spray the pan again with oil and return to medium heat. Add the garlic and ginger and cook, stirring, for 1 minute. Add the veggie noodles, along with a small splash of hot water to create steam. Stir-fry for 2–3 minutes or until just tender.

4. Divide the noodles and patties among plates, scatter over the coriander leaves and serve.

307	9.3 g
Calories	Carbs

Nutritional Information
(per serve)

Calories	**307**
Protein	**31.3 g**
Fat Total	**14.8 g**
Fat Saturated	**4.0 g**
Carbohydrates	**9.3 g**
Sugars	**8.7 g**
Sodium	**375.4 mg**
Dietary Fibre	**7.3 g**

Mish Tips

You can buy pre-made veggie noodles, or use a spiraliser. Alternatively, cut the carrot and zucchini with a julienne peeler or regular veggie peeler into ribbons. You don't have to use yellow curry paste for this; if you prefer a different type of curry paste, go right ahead.

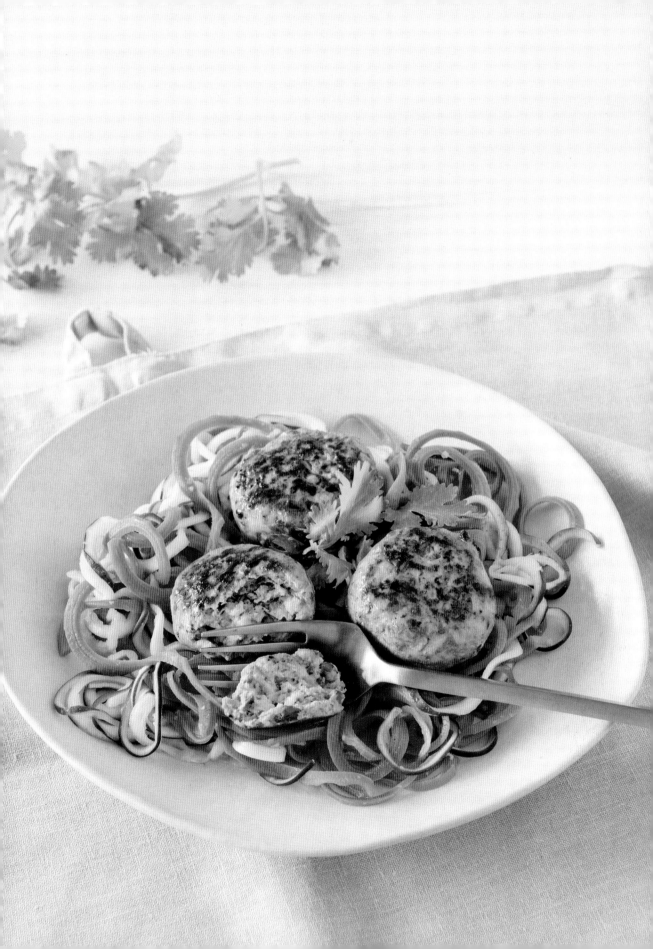

Miso salmon with cauliflower fried rice

Cauliflower fried rice will change your low-carb life — get into it!
Use it anywhere you'd normally have rice.

Serves: **2** · Prep time: **10 minutes** · Cooking time: **10 minutes** · Great for: *Dinner*

Ingredients

200 g Atlantic salmon fillet, skin and
    bones removed
1 tablespoon miso soybean paste
1 teaspoon honey
250 g cauliflower, cut into florets
1 teaspoon olive oil
3 spring onions, finely sliced, white
    and green parts separated
1 teaspoon finely grated ginger
1 clove garlic, crushed
⅓ cup frozen peas, thawed
2 teaspoons salt-reduced soy sauce
2 tablespoons chopped coriander
½ lime, cut into wedges

Method

1. Cut the salmon into two equal portions. Combine the miso paste and honey and rub all over the salmon. Place on a baking tray lined with foil and set aside.

2. Preheat the grill to medium–high. Cook the salmon under the grill for 4 minutes each side.

3. Meanwhile, place the cauliflower in a food processor and blitz until it resembles grains of rice. Heat the olive oil in a wok or deep non-stick frying pan over medium heat. Add the cauliflower, white part of the spring onion, ginger and garlic and stir-fry for 5 minutes or until tender. Add the peas and stir-fry for a further 3 minutes or until tender. Toss through the soy sauce.

4. Divide the cauliflower rice and salmon between plates and sprinkle with the coriander and green part of the spring onion. Serve with the lime wedges on the side.

308	**9.8** g
Calories	Carbs

Nutritional Information

(per serve)

Calories	**308**
Protein	**26.5 g**
Fat Total	**16.9 g**
Fat Saturated	**4.2 g**
Carbohydrates	**9.8 g**
Sugars	**7.1 g**
Sodium	**789.0 mg**
Dietary Fibre	**6.6 g**

Mish Tips

Make sure the salmon isn't too close to the heat source under the grill, otherwise it will burn. The rack should be about 10 cm from the heat.

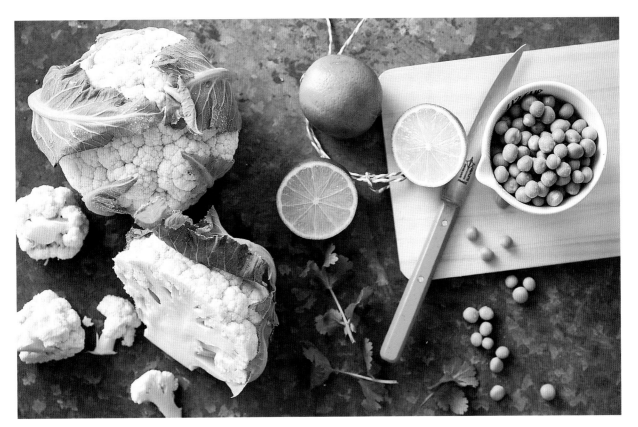

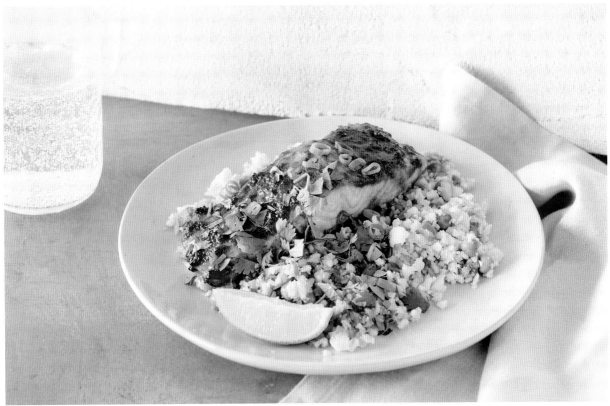

Veggie and tofu tray bake with feta cream

Vego meals can often be high in carbs, but not this one! Try this delicious vegetarian option for Meatless Mondays, Tuesdays, Wednesdays . . .

Serves: **4** · Prep time: **20 minutes** · Cooking time: **40 minutes** · Great for: *Dinner*

Ingredients

300 g cauliflower, cut into florets
2 bunches broccolini, trimmed and
    halved lengthways
400 g firm tofu, sliced
4 carrots, quartered lengthways
olive oil spray
1 tablespoon dukkah
70 g kale, stalks removed, leaves torn
¾ cup low-fat natural yoghurt
60 g low-fat feta, mashed
2 cloves garlic, crushed
1 tablespoon tahini

Method

1. Preheat the oven to 190°C (170°C fan-forced). Line two large baking trays with baking paper. Arrange the cauliflower, broccolini, tofu and carrot over the trays and lightly spray with olive oil. Sprinkle with the dukkah and season well with freshly ground black pepper. Bake for 30 minutes.

2. Add the kale and bake for a further 10 minutes or until lightly crisp and the veggies are tender and golden.

3. Meanwhile, place the yoghurt, feta, garlic and tahini in a small bowl and mix well.

4. Divide the baked tofu and vegetables among plates and serve with the feta cream.

304 / 8.4 g
Calories / Carbs

Nutritional Information
(per serve)

Calories	**304**
Protein	**26.4 g**
Fat Total	**14.8 g**
Fat Saturated	**4.4 g**
Carbohydrates	**8.4 g**
Sugars	**8.1 g**
Sodium	**317.0 mg**
Dietary Fibre	**16.1 g**

Mish Tips

Dukkah is an Egyptian spice mix of dried herbs, sesame seeds, nuts and spices. Look for it in the spice section of your supermarket. If you can't find it, use a blend of equal parts sesame seeds and ground cumin.

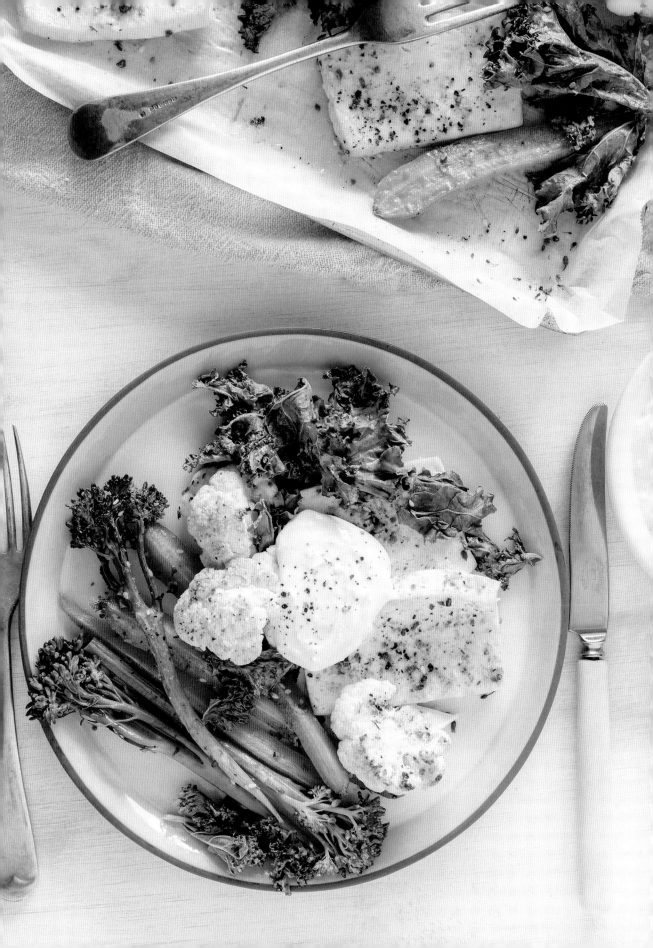

Warm *chicken* salad

This recipe is sure to impress anyone you make it for. It's easy to double or triple the recipe, making it a great option to have in your back pocket for your next family gathering.

Serves: **2** • Prep time: **10 minutes** • Cooking time: **5 minutes** • Great for: *Lunch*

324 Calories   **6.1 g** Carbs

Ingredients

2 teaspoons olive oil
150 g green beans, trimmed
  and chopped
110 g asparagus, trimmed and chopped
100 g brussels sprouts, trimmed and
  finely shredded
250 g cooked lean chicken breast
  fillet, shredded
1 tablespoon desiccated coconut
1 teaspoon pumpkin seeds
½ cup mint leaves, torn
2 tablespoons buttermilk
1 tablespoon lemon juice

Method

1. Heat the olive oil in a large non-stick frying pan over medium heat. Add the beans and asparagus and stir-fry for 2 minutes or until tender-crisp. Add the brussels sprouts and toss for 1 minute or until just softened.

2. Remove the pan from the heat and add the chicken, coconut, pumpkin seeds and mint. Season with freshly ground black pepper and toss to combine. Divide between two bowls.

3. Whisk together the buttermilk and lemon juice in a small jug. Drizzle over the salad bowls and serve.

Nutritional Information
(per serve)

Calories	**324**
Protein	**44.2 g**
Fat Total	**12.2 g**
Fat Saturated	**4.2 g**
Carbohydrates	**6.1 g**
Sugars	**4.6 g**
Sodium	**85.3 mg**
Dietary Fibre	**6.8 g**

Mish Tips

To cook the chicken, poach a breast fillet in a saucepan of gently simmering water for 10–15 minutes or until cooked through. Cool, then pack into an airtight container and store in the fridge for up to 3 days. Alternatively, use a barbecue chicken with the skin removed.

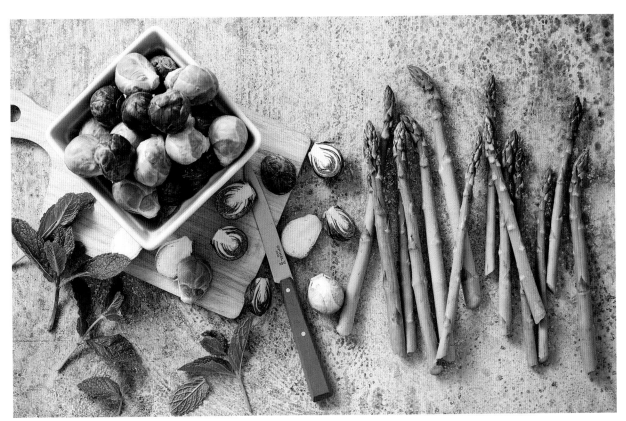

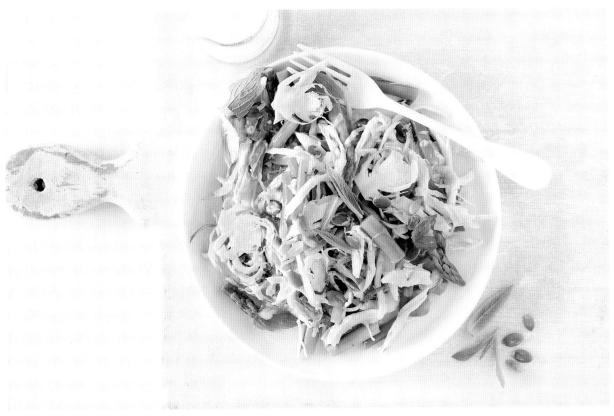

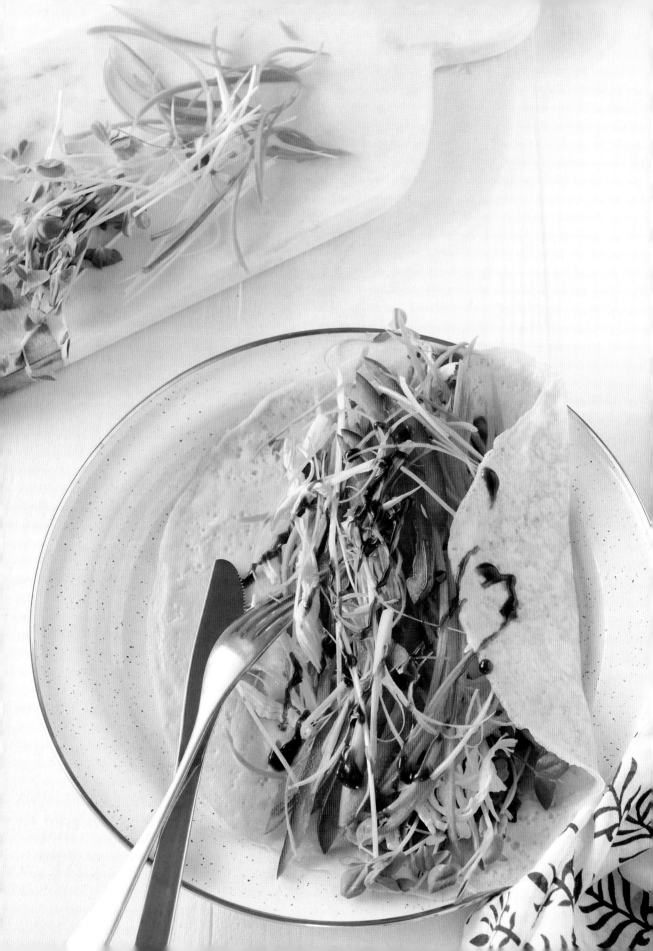

Asian chicken omelette

Oh, I love an omelette! So quick and easy, and this one has a yummy Asian aspect to it.

Serves: **2** · Prep time: **10 minutes** · Cooking time: **5 minutes** · Great for: *Breakfast, Lunch or Dinner*

Ingredients

olive oil spray

4 cage-free eggs

35 g snow pea sprouts

125 g cooked lean chicken breast fillet, shredded

1 red capsicum, seeded and finely sliced

1 carrot, grated

1 spring onion, shredded

3 teaspoons oyster sauce

Method

1. Lightly spray a wok or large non-stick frying pan with olive oil and heat over medium–high heat. Whisk the eggs and 1 tablespoon water in a bowl. Pour half the egg mixture into the wok and swirl to coat the base. Cook for 2 minutes or until the egg has almost set.

2. Slide the omelette onto a serving plate and arrange half the snow pea sprouts, chicken, capsicum, carrot and spring onion in the centre. Fold or roll up the omelette to enclose the filling. Repeat with the remaining ingredients to make a second omelette. Drizzle the omelettes with oyster sauce and serve.

302	7.1 g
Calories	Carbs

Nutritional Information
(per serve)

Calories	**302**
Protein	**35.8 g**
Fat Total	**14.1 g**
Fat Saturated	**3.8 g**
Carbohydrates	**7.1 g**
Sugars	**6.4 g**
Sodium	**484.8 mg**
Dietary Fibre	**2.7 g**

Mish Tips

To cook the chicken, poach a breast fillet in a saucepan of gently simmering water for 10–15 minutes or until cooked through. Cool, then pack into an airtight container and store in the fridge for up to 3 days. Alternatively, use a barbecue chicken with the skin removed.

Grilled fish with herbed veggie 'couscous'

Grilled fish is a staple for me, and I love this creative take on 'couscous'. It only takes 15 minutes to whip up this zesty meal.

Serves: **1** • Prep time: **10 minutes** • Cooking time: **5 minutes** • Great for: *Dinner*

Ingredients

1 zucchini, trimmed and roughly chopped
75 g broccoli, stalks included, roughly chopped
15 g unsalted pistachio kernels
½ clove garlic, peeled
1 tablespoon chopped mint
1 tablespoon chopped coriander
½ lemon, zest finely grated, lemon cut into wedges
1 teaspoon extra virgin olive oil
150 g white fish fillet, skin and bones removed
olive oil spray

Method

1. Place the zucchini, broccoli, pistachios and garlic in a food processor and pulse just until finely chopped. Transfer the mixture to a bowl and add the mint, coriander and lemon zest. Drizzle with the extra virgin olive oil, season well with freshly ground black pepper and toss to combine.

2. Preheat the grill to medium–high. Place the fish on a baking tray, lightly spray with olive oil, and season with freshly ground black pepper. Cook the fish under the grill for 2 minutes each side or until cooked through.

3. Scoop the veggie 'couscous' onto a plate, add the fish and serve with the lemon wedges on the side.

307	**4.1** g
Calories	Carbs

Nutritional Information
(per serve)

Calories	**307**
Protein	**31.3 g**
Fat Total	**17.0 g**
Fat Saturated	**2.5 g**
Carbohydrates	**4.1 g**
Sugars	**3.8 g**
Sodium	**20.9 m**
Dietary Fibre	**6.9 g**

Mish Tips

The cooking time may vary, depending on the type and thickness of the fish you use. If you are using frozen fish, let it thaw completely before cooking. The olive oil in the 'couscous' adds to the flavour so make sure you use a good-quality one.

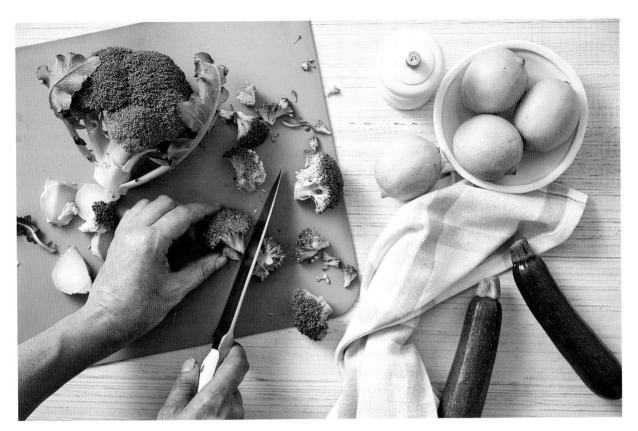

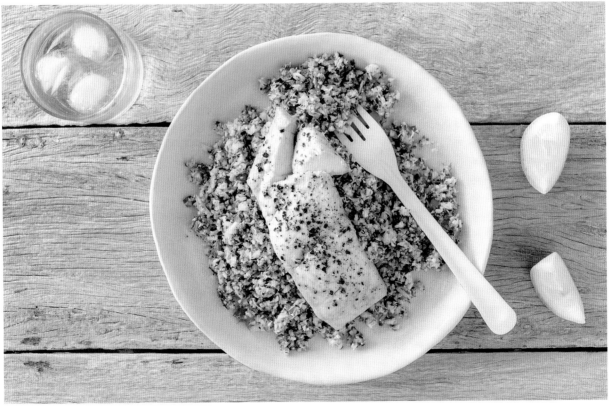

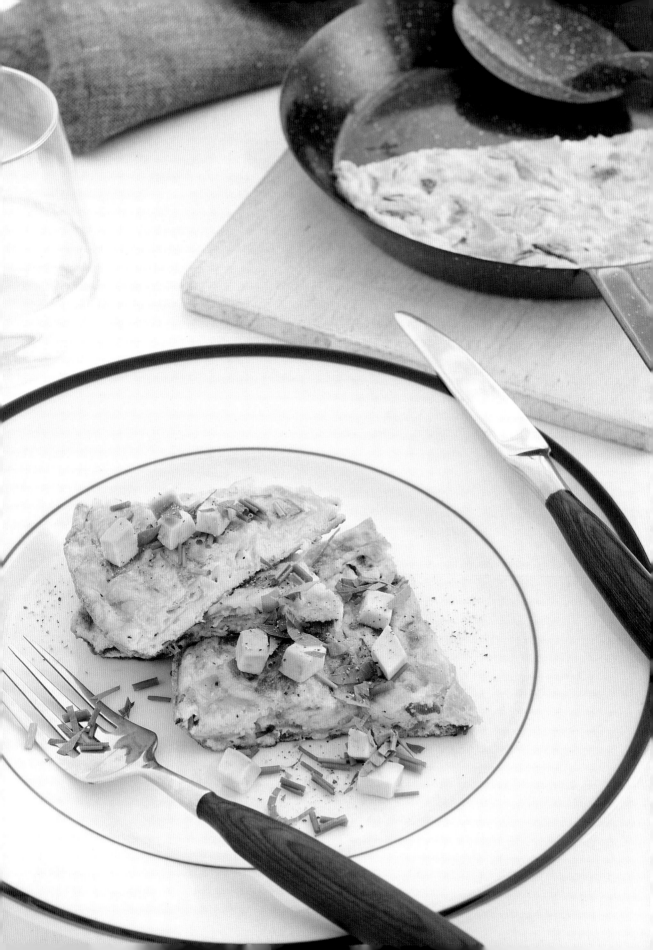

Roasted capsicum and ham frittata with avocado and herb salad

Frittatas are a great way to reduce food waste as you can use whatever fresh vegetables and herbs you have in your crisper. We have them loads in our household.

Serves: **2** · Prep time: **15 minutes** · Cooking time: **15 minutes** · Great for: *Breakfast or Lunch*

339	2.8 g
Calories	Carbs

Ingredients

3 cage-free eggs
2 cage-free egg whites
70 g lean ham, chopped
70 g chargrilled capsicum, chopped
40 g low-fat cheddar, grated
1 tablespoon finely chopped chives
olive oil spray
60 g avocado, diced
1 tablespoon finely chopped
flat-leaf parsley

Method

1. Whisk together the eggs and egg whites in a bowl. Add the ham, capsicum, cheddar and half the chives and stir to combine.

2. Lightly spray a small (20 cm) non-stick frying pan with olive oil and heat over low heat. Add the egg mixture, then cover and cook for 10 minutes or until almost set.

3. Meanwhile, combine the avocado, parsley and the remaining chives in a small bowl and season with freshly ground black pepper.

4. Preheat the grill to high. Grill the frittata for 5 minutes or until golden, puffed and set. Cut into wedges and serve warm with the avocado salad.

Nutritional Information
(per serve)

Calories	**339**
Protein	**27.5 g**
Fat Total	**23.9 g**
Fat Saturated	**7.5 g**
Carbohydrates	**2.8 g**
Sugars	**1.4 g**
Sodium	**829.3 mg**
Dietary Fibre	**1.6 g**

Mish Tips

To chargrill a capsicum, cut it into large pieces and remove the seeds and membrane. Place, skin side up, under a hot grill or, skin side down, on a hot chargrill pan and cook until the skin has blistered and blackened. Let it cool, then remove the skin and cut the flesh as required. Protect the handle of your frying pan with a damp tea towel while grilling. Take care as it will get hot. Leftover frittata is delicious served for lunch with mixed salad leaves.

Fish kebabs with green leaf salad

A fun fish twist on the classic kebab. These flavours also work really well with chicken, tofu or prawns, so it's a really versatile little recipe!

Serves: **2** · Prep time: **20 minutes** · Cooking time: **5 minutes** · Great for: *Dinner*

323
Calories

4.6 g
Carbs

Ingredients

200 g white fish fillets, skin and bones removed, cut into 2 cm chunks

200 g Atlantic salmon fillets, skin and bones removed, cut into 2 cm chunks

finely grated zest and juice of 1 lemon

½ brown onion, finely chopped

1 tablespoon chopped dill

1 clove garlic, crushed

1 teaspoon finely grated ginger

olive oil spray

70 g baby spinach leaves

1 celery stalk, leaves on, sliced

Method

1. Combine the white fish, salmon, lemon zest, onion, dill, garlic and ginger in a large bowl. Season well with freshly ground black pepper and toss to combine.

2. Thread the white fish and salmon alternately onto four skewers.

3. Heat a chargrill pan over medium–high heat. Lightly spray the skewers with olive oil and cook for 5 minutes, turning often, until the fish is lightly golden and cooked through. (Alternatively, cook on a foil-lined baking tray under a hot grill for 8–10 minutes.)

4. Meanwhile, toss the spinach leaves, celery and celery leaves in a bowl.

5. Divide the salad between plates, add the skewers and finish with a squeeze of lemon juice.

Nutritional Information
(per serve)

Calories	**323**
Protein	**38.7 g**
Fat Total	**16.0 g**
Fat Saturated	**4.3 g**
Carbohydrates	**4.6 g**
Sugars	**3.3 g**
Sodium	**103.3 mg**
Dietary Fibre	**3.6 g**

Mish Tips

If you are using wooden or bamboo skewers, soak them in cold water for 15 minutes before threading the fish on, to prevent them burning during cooking. A handful of fresh rocket would be a delicious addition to the salad mix.

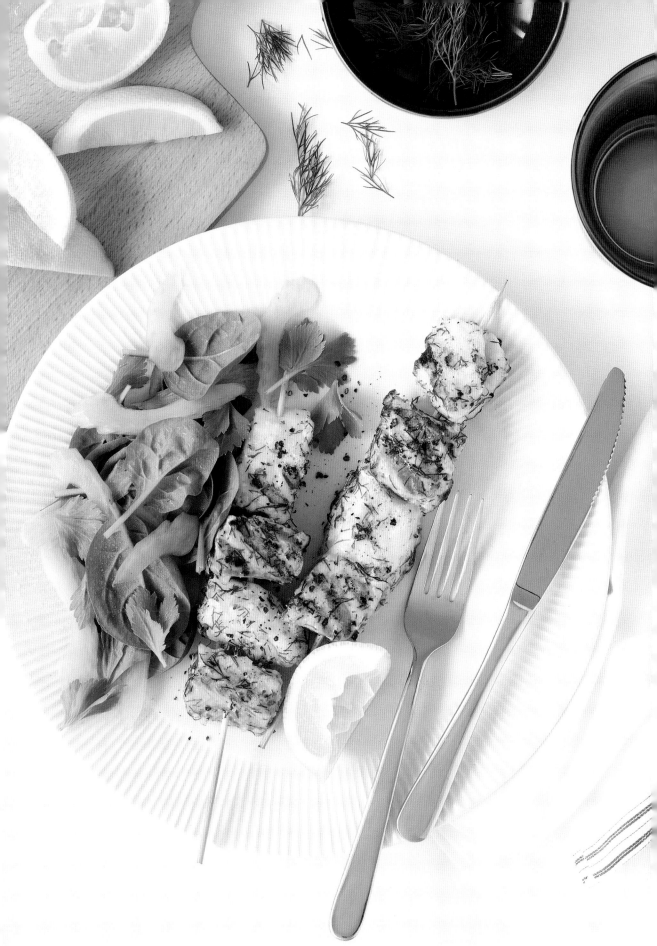

Chicken kebabs with radish and cucumber salad

Fun, fast and easy, kebabs are a meal the kids can help to create, and they'll love eating the results! The Japanese flavours make these a favourite for us. Get the chicken marinating the night before for extra flavour.

Serves: **2** · Prep time: **15 minutes, plus 30 minutes chilling** · Cooking time: **10 minutes** ·
Great for: *Weekend Lunch*

310	2.7 g
Calories	Carbs

Ingredients

2 tablespoons salt-reduced soy sauce

2 tablespoons mirin

2 tablespoons rice wine vinegar

2 cloves garlic, crushed

300 g lean chicken breast fillet, cut into chunks

olive oil spray

75 g iceberg lettuce, torn

3 radishes, trimmed and finely sliced

1 Lebanese cucumber, finely sliced

Method

1. Combine the soy sauce, mirin, rice wine vinegar and garlic in a shallow non-metallic dish. Take out 1 tablespoon of the marinade and reserve. Add the chicken to the dish and turn to coat, then cover and refrigerate for 30 minutes, or longer if time permits.

2. Preheat a barbecue grill or flat plate to medium. Thread the chicken onto six skewers and lightly spray with olive oil. Cook, turning occasionally, for 8–10 minutes or until the chicken is golden brown and cooked through.

3. Meanwhile, toss the lettuce, radish and cucumber in a bowl and drizzle with the reserved marinade. Serve with the skewers.

Nutritional Information

(per serve)

Calories	**310**
Protein	**35.7 g**
Fat Total	**17.5 g**
Fat Saturated	**7.6 g**
Carbohydrates	**2.7 g**
Sugars	**2.2 g**
Sodium	**754.5 mg**
Dietary Fibre	**1.9 g**

Mish Tips

Iceberg lettuce works best in this dish but other types of lettuce are also fine if that's what you have. If you are using wooden or bamboo skewers, soak them in cold water for 15 minutes before threading the chicken on, to prevent them burning during cooking.

Mushroom omelettes with spinach and cherry tomatoes

It's amazing that something so lean can taste like such a treat. This omelette is a substantial meal that will leave you feeling super satisfied.

Serves: **2** · Prep time: **15 minutes** · Cooking time: **25 minutes** · Great for: *Breakfast*

Ingredients

olive oil spray

½ red onion, finely sliced

200 g mushrooms, quartered

3 cage-free eggs

3 cage-free egg whites

180 g low-fat cottage cheese

20 g baby spinach leaves

250 g cherry tomatoes, halved

1 tablespoon lemon juice

Method

1. Lightly spray a large ovenproof frying pan with olive oil and heat over medium heat. Add the onion and cook for 4 minutes or until golden. Transfer to a bowl. Add the mushroom to the pan and cook for 4 minutes or until lightly browned. Add to the onion.

2. Place the eggs and egg whites in a large bowl and beat until fluffy. Using a large metal spoon, fold in the mushroom and onion mixture.

3. Lightly spray the pan with olive oil again and reheat over medium–low heat. Preheat the grill to medium.

4. Pour half the omelette mixture into the pan and gently tilt to cover the base. Cook for 4 minutes or until almost set.

5. Place the pan under the grill for 3 minutes or until the top is set. Transfer to a plate and cover with foil to keep warm. Repeat with the remaining omelette mixture.

6. Spread the cottage cheese over the omelettes and top with spinach leaves and tomatoes. Gently roll up to enclose the filling. Season with freshly ground black pepper and drizzle with the lemon juice, then serve immediately.

324 Calories   **7.8** g Carbs

Nutritional Information
(per serve)

Calories	**324**
Protein	**35.6 g**
Fat Total	**14.9 g**
Fat Saturated	**5.6 g**
Carbohydrates	**7.8 g**
Sugars	**7.5 g**
Sodium	**488.4 mg**
Dietary Fibre	**4.7 g**

Mish Tips

There is nothing worse than an overcooked omelette so keep an eye on it under the grill.

Prosciutto-wrapped chicken with wilted greens

Did someone say chicken wrapped in bacon? Yes please! We use prosciutto here, but if you happen to have bacon in your fridge, you can use that instead.

Serves: **2** • Prep time: **15 minutes** • Cooking time: **25 minutes** • Great for: *Dinner*

Ingredients

2 x 150 g lean chicken breast fillets
2 teaspoons dijon mustard
30 g prosciutto, finely sliced
2 teaspoons olive oil
½ bunch English spinach, trimmed
    and halved crossways
2 cloves garlic, finely sliced
60 g kale, stalks removed, leaves torn
1 lemon, halved

Method

1. Preheat the oven to 180°C (160°C fan-forced). Line a baking tray with baking paper.

2. Place the chicken on the prepared tray and spread the mustard over the chicken. Drape the prosciutto over the fillets and tuck in the edges. Bake for 20–25 minutes or until tender and cooked through.

3. Meanwhile, heat the olive oil in a large non-stick frying pan over medium heat. Add the spinach and garlic and stir-fry for 30 seconds. Add the kale and stir-fry for a further 1–2 minutes or until the greens are just wilted. Squeeze the juice from one lemon half over the top and toss to combine.

4. Cut the chicken into thick slices. Divide the wilted greens between two plates, top with the chicken and season with freshly ground black pepper. Cut the remaining lemon half into wedges and serve on the side.

288 Calories   3.3 g Carbs

Nutritional Information
(per serve)

Calories	**288**
Protein	**41.2 g**
Fat Total	**10.5 g**
Fat Saturated	**2.5 g**
Carbohydrates	**3.3 g**
Sugars	**2.5 g**
Sodium	**578.5 mg**
Dietary Fibre	**6.1 g**

Mish Tips

Try replacing the spinach and kale with Asian greens, such as bok choy or Chinese broccoli (gai lan).

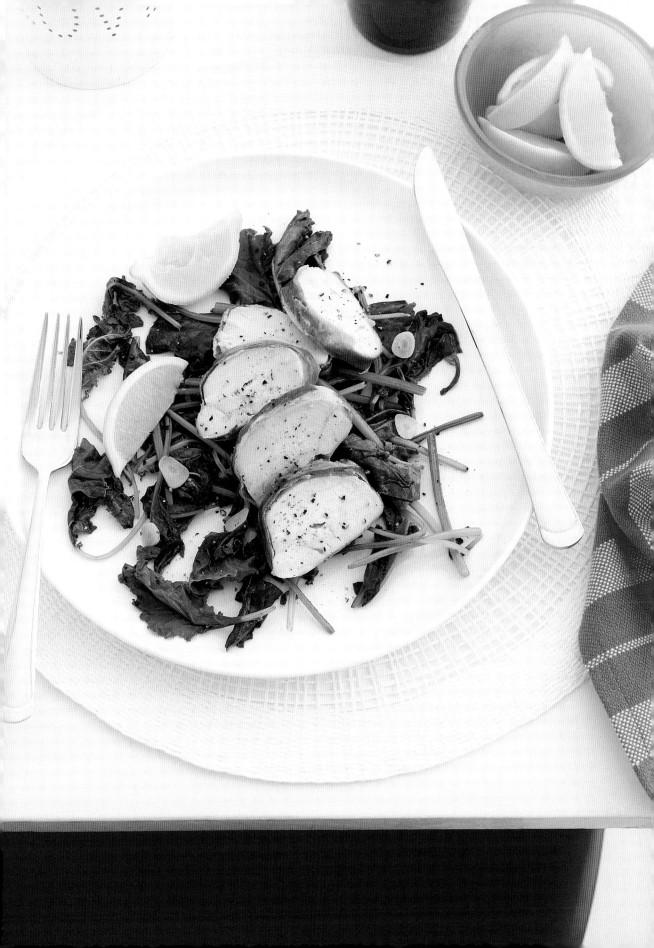

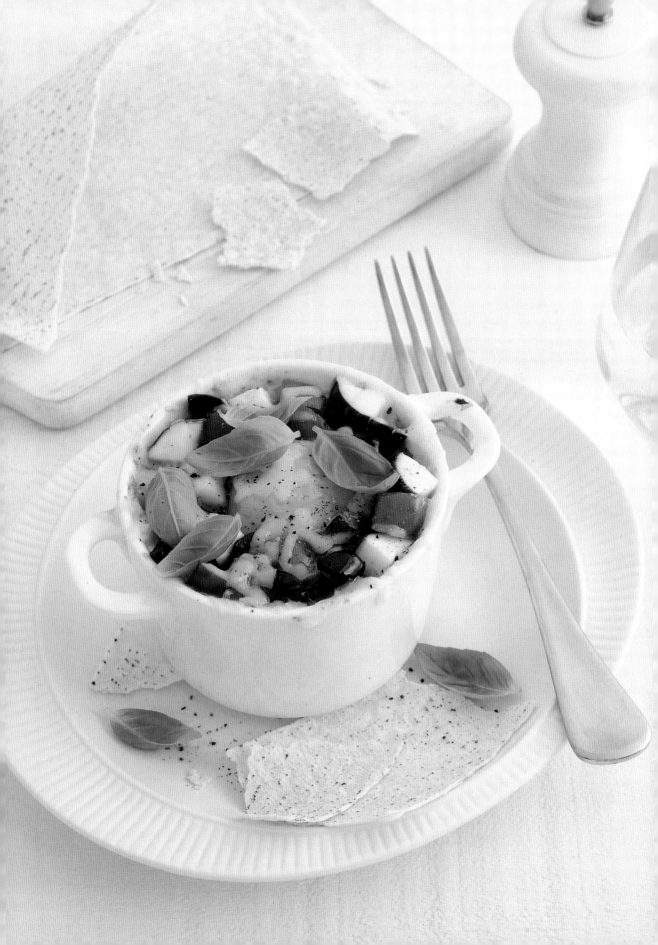

Italian–style baked eggs

Baked eggs is one of my favourite ways to eat eggs, and this recipe is full of flavour. The soft eggs are paired with classic Italian ingredients, such as tomatoes, olives and basil.

Serves: **2** · Prep time: **15 minutes** · Cooking time: **30 minutes** · Great for: *Breakfast*

294	7.1 g
Calories	Carbs

Ingredients

2 tomatoes, chopped

1 zucchini, finely chopped

½ red capsicum, seeded and finely chopped

1 clove garlic, crushed

1 teaspoon olive oil

8 kalamata olives, pitted

4 cage-free eggs

20 g low-fat cheddar, grated

3 tablespoons baby basil leaves

Method

1. Preheat the oven to 190°C (170°C fan-forced). Line a large baking tray with baking paper.

2. Scatter the tomato, zucchini, capsicum and garlic over the prepared tray. Drizzle with the olive oil and toss to coat, then roast for 20 minutes or until almost tender. Remove from the oven. Reduce the temperature to 180°C (160°C fan-forced).

3. Toss the olives through the vegetables and divide half between two small baking dishes. Make an indentation in each dish. Crack an egg into each indentation and sprinkle with the cheese. Repeat with the remaining vegetable mixture, eggs and cheese.

4. Bake for 8–10 minutes or until the egg whites are set and the yolks are still runny. Scatter over the basil leaves, season with freshly ground black pepper and serve.

Nutritional Information

(per serve)

Calories	**294**
Protein	**21.0 g**
Fat Total	**19.5 g**
Fat Saturated	**5.5 g**
Carbohydrates	**7.1 g**
Sugars	**6.4 g**
Sodium	**405.2 mg**
Dietary Fibre	**4.2 g**

Less than 10 grams of carbs

Oven-roasted lamb rack with tomatoes and salsa verde

Lamb is super high in nutrition and this recipe is super high in flavour. It's perfect for a special occasion or large dinner party. Enjoy!

Serves: **10** • Prep time: **25 minutes** • Cooking time: **35 minutes** • Great for: *Weekend Lunch or Dinner*

Ingredients

1.2 kg frenched lamb racks
750 g cherry tomatoes
olive oil spray
8 kalamata olives, pitted
1 tablespoon olive oil
1 clove garlic, roughly chopped
½ cup coriander leaves
½ cup flat-leaf parsley leaves
1 anchovy fillet
2 teaspoons white balsamic vinegar
300 g mixed salad leaves

Method

1. Preheat the oven to 200°C (180°C fan-forced). Line a large baking dish with baking paper.

2. Place the lamb racks in the prepared dish and scatter the tomatoes around the lamb. Lightly spray with olive oil and season with freshly ground black pepper. Roast for 10 minutes, then reduce the temperature to 180°C (160°C fan-forced) and roast for a further 20–25 minutes for medium, or until cooked to your liking.

3. Remove from the oven, cover loosely with foil and rest for 10 minutes.

4. Meanwhile, combine the olives, olive oil, garlic, coriander, parsley, anchovy, vinegar and 3 tablespoons water in a large jug. Blend with a hand-held blender until smooth.

5. Slice the lamb, allowing two cutlets per person. Arrange the cutlets and tomatoes on plates, drizzle with the salsa verde and serve with the salad leaves.

241	2.4 g
Calories	Carbs

Nutritional Information
(per serve)

Calories	**241**
Protein	**26.9 g**
Fat Total	**13.4 g**
Fat Saturated	**4.5 g**
Carbohydrates	**2.4 g**
Sugars	**2.2 g**
Sodium	**163.8 mg**
Dietary Fibre	**2.0 g**

Mish Tips

Use a combination of red and yellow tomatoes for a festive look, or just red if that's what you have to hand. 'Frenched' means all the fat has been trimmed from the lamb and the bones have been scraped clean for an attractive presentation. You can generally buy them like that, or ask your butcher to do it for you.

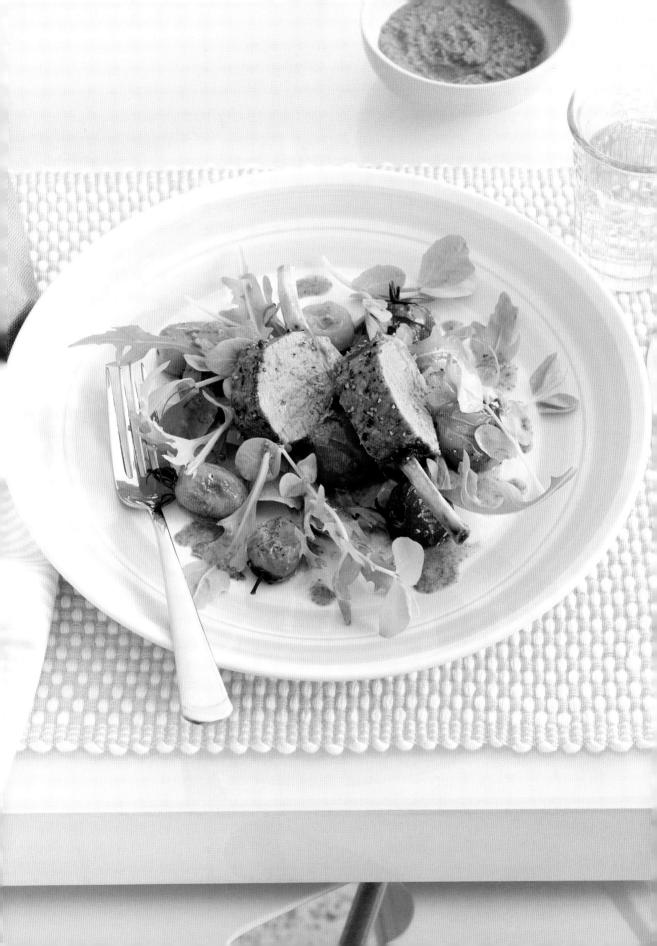

Japanese tofu and cabbage pancake

Is it an omelette or a pancake? Who cares, when it tastes so good? Japanese cuisine has it covered — clean, tasty eats that won't break the calorie bank.

Serves: **2** • Prep time: **15 minutes** • Cooking time: **25 minutes** • Great for: *Breakfast or Lunch*

Ingredients

1 teaspoon sesame oil

250 g Chinese cabbage (wombok), shredded

3 spring onions, finely sliced

2 teaspoons salt-reduced soy sauce

2 teaspoons finely grated ginger

150 g firm tofu, chopped

4 cage-free eggs

olive oil spray

2 teaspoons oyster sauce

½ sheet nori, cut into strips

Method

1. Heat the sesame oil in a large non-stick frying pan over medium heat and swirl to coat the base. Add the cabbage and cook, stirring, for 2–3 minutes or until almost wilted.

2. Add most of the spring onion (save a bit for garnish) and cook, stirring, for a further 2 minutes or until softened. Remove from the heat and set aside to cool. Whisk together the soy sauce, ginger, tofu and eggs in a large bowl, then stir through the cooled cabbage mixture.

3. Lightly spray a small non-stick frying pan with olive oil and heat over medium heat. Spoon one-quarter of the cabbage mixture into the pan and spread over the base. Cook for 2–3 minutes each side or until golden and cooked through. Remove to a plate and cover to keep warm. Repeat with the remaining mixture to make four pancakes in total.

4. Divide the pancakes between two plates. Drizzle with the oyster sauce, top with the nori and reserved spring onion and serve.

314	3.5 g
Calories	Carbs

Nutritional Information

(per serve)

Calories	**314**
Protein	**26.6 g**
Fat Total	**20.3 g**
Fat Saturated	**4.5 g**
Carbohydrates	**3.5 g**
Sugars	**3.0 g**
Sodium	**728.8 mg**
Dietary Fibre	**7.0 g**

Mish Tips

To make this dish vegetarian, replace the oyster sauce with kecap manis or hoisin sauce.

Quick prawn curry

I love curry, seafood and quick meals, and this delicious recipe ticks all the boxes. This is not a hot curry but you could add some fresh chilli if you like things spicy.

Serves: **2** · Prep time: **15 minutes** · Cooking time: **10 minutes** · Great for: *Dinner*

297	5.7 g
Calories	Carbs

Ingredients

1 tablespoon olive oil

1 clove garlic, crushed

3 teaspoons korma curry paste

160 g raw king prawns, peeled and deveined

200 g low-fat coconut milk

200 g Chinese broccoli (gai lan), chopped

1 zucchini, chopped

100 g green beans, trimmed and chopped

1 tablespoon lightly dried coriander

Method

1. Heat the olive oil in a wok or large non-stick frying pan over medium–high heat. Add the garlic and curry paste and cook, stirring, for 30 seconds or until fragrant. Add the prawns and toss to coat in the spice mix.

2. Pour in the coconut milk and bring to a simmer. Add the Chinese broccoli and zucchini, then cover and simmer for 2 minutes. Add the beans and simmer, covered, for a further 2–3 minutes or until the vegetables are just cooked through. Stir through the coriander.

3. Divide the curry between bowls and serve.

Nutritional Information
(per serve)

Calories	**297**
Protein	**21.6 g**
Fat Total	**19.3 g**
Fat Saturated	**8.4 g**
Carbohydrates	**5.7 g**
Sugars	**4.4 g**
Sodium	**411.8 mg**
Dietary Fibre	**2.9 g**

Mish Tips

If preferred, you can use thawed frozen prawns for this recipe. Look for 'lightly dried' coriander in the fresh fruit and veg aisle at the supermarket. It has great flavour and colour. Alternatively, sprinkle over some fresh coriander at the end.

Seared salmon with vegetable noodles

Vegetable noodles are a great way to lower your carbs without losing that satisfying 'full' feeling after your meal.

Serves: **2** • Prep time: **5 minutes** • Cooking time: **10 minutes** • Great for: *Dinner*

Ingredients

1 teaspoon salt-reduced soy sauce

1 teaspoon sesame oil

200 g Atlantic salmon fillet, skin and bones removed

olive oil spray

2 carrots, cut into noodles

3 zucchini, cut into noodles

40 g baby spinach leaves

1 teaspoon sweet chilli sauce

Method

1. Combine the soy sauce and sesame oil in a bowl, then add the salmon and turn to coat. Lightly spray a non-stick frying pan with olive oil and heat over medium–high heat. Add the salmon and cook for 2–3 minutes each side (depending on thickness) or until just cooked through. Remove from the heat and set aside on a plate. Wipe out the pan.

2. Lightly spray the pan with olive oil again and place over medium heat. Add the shredded vegetables and stir-fry, adding a tiny splash of hot water to create steam, for 2 minutes or until just tender.

3. Scatter over the spinach and cook for 1 minute or until just wilted. Add the chilli sauce and toss to combine.

4. Divide the vegetable mixture between bowls, top with the salmon and serve.

276	6.8 g
Calories	Carbs

Nutritional Information
(per serve)

Calories	**276**
Protein	**23.2 g**
Fat Total	**17.0 g**
Fat Saturated	**4.2 g**
Carbohydrates	**6.8 g**
Sugars	**6.0 g**
Sodium	**281.1 mg**
Dietary Fibre	**4.8 g**

Mish Tips

You can use a veggie spiraliser for the zucchini and carrot if you have one. Alternatively, you can buy a small shredder (which looks a bit like a veggie peeler). Both are available in kitchenware shops, and are inexpensive and easy to use.

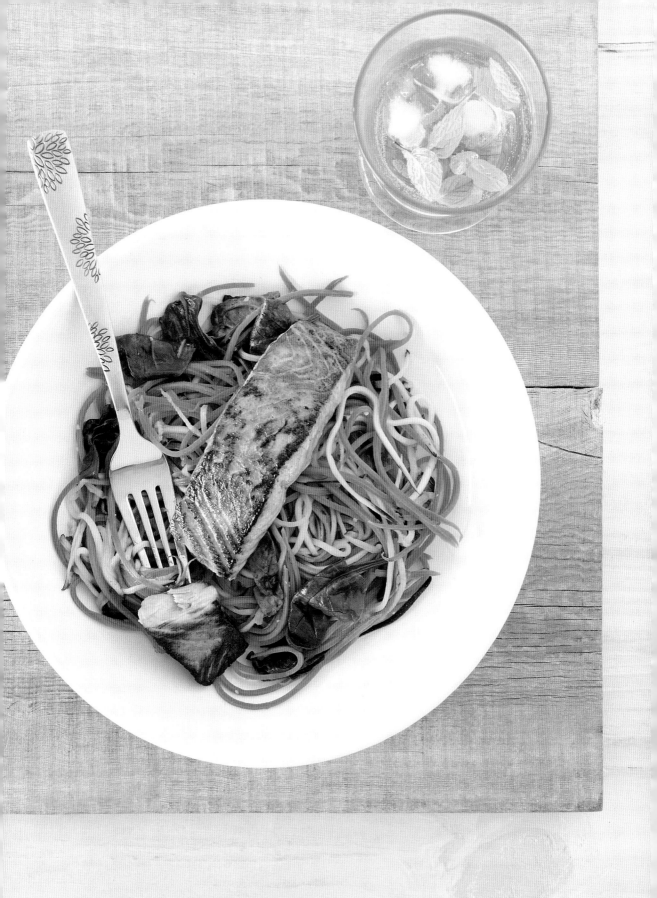

Steak with creamy mushroom sauce

Everyone loves a creamy sauce on their steak. This mushroom and garlic sauce tastes so decadent but is certainly not a disaster for your waistline. Give it a go!

Serves: **2** · Prep time: **15 minutes** · Cooking time: **10 minutes** · Great for: *Dinner*

Ingredients

olive oil spray
2 x 140 g lean rump steaks
½ brown onion, sliced
2 cloves garlic, crushed
200 g mushrooms, sliced
80 g extra light cream cheese
2 carrots, cut into sticks
1 bunch broccolini, trimmed

Method

1. Lightly spray a non-stick frying pan with olive oil and heat over medium–high heat. Add the steaks and cook for 2 minutes each side for medium, or until cooked to your liking. Transfer to a plate, cover with foil and set aside to rest.

2. Spray the pan with a little more oil. Add the onion and garlic and cook, stirring often, for 2–3 minutes or until softened. Add the mushroom and cook, stirring often, for 2–3 minutes or until tender. Dollop in the cream cheese and stir slowly until a sauce forms, adding a little water if necessary. Season with freshly ground black pepper.

3. Meanwhile, cook the carrot and broccolini in a steamer set over a saucepan of simmering water for 2 minutes or until tender.

4. Divide the steaks, carrot and broccolini between two plates. Spoon the sauce over the steaks and serve.

308 Calories   7.6 g Carbs

Nutritional Information
(per serve)

Calories	**308**
Protein	**40.9 g**
Fat Total	**9.6 g**
Fat Saturated	**3.8 g**
Carbohydrates	**7.6 g**
Sugars	**7.3 g**
Sodium	**232.2 mg**
Dietary Fibre	**8.1 g**

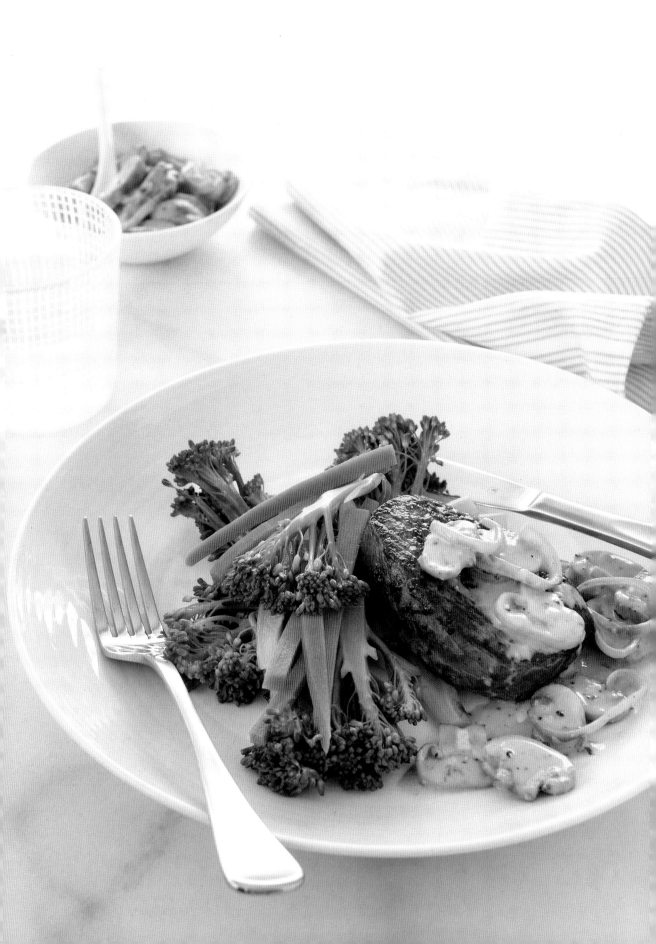

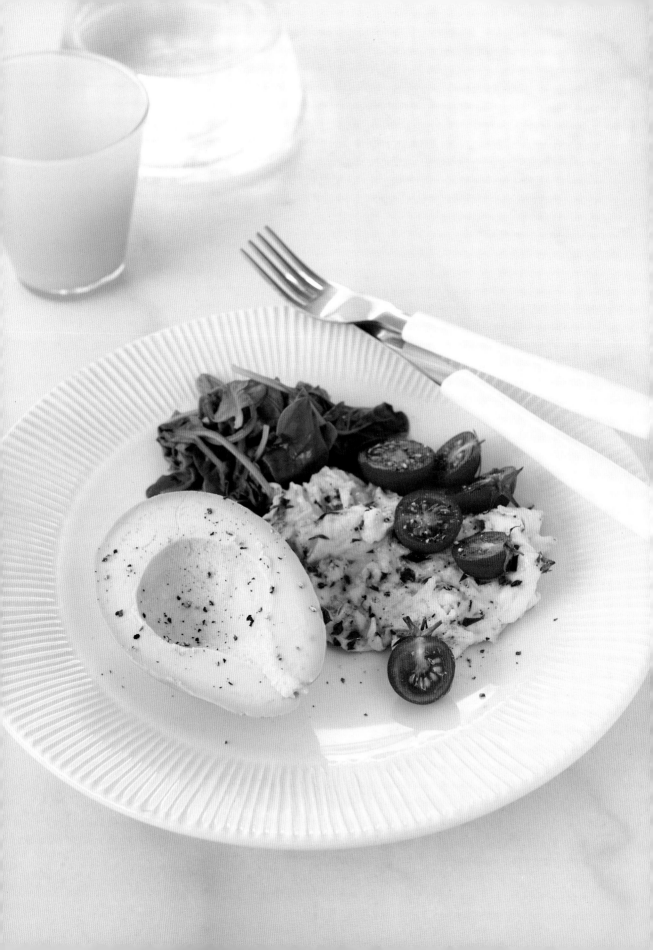

Scrambled eggs with spinach and avocado

Eggs with two of my favourite greens? Why, I don't mind if I do!

Serves: **2** • Prep time: **15 minutes** • Cooking time: **5 minutes** • Great for: *Breakfast*

Ingredients

2 cage-free eggs

2 cage-free egg whites

2 tablespoons chopped
    flat-leaf parsley

olive oil spray

80 g baby spinach leaves

boiling water, for blanching

1 avocado, halved

125 g cherry tomatoes, halved

Method

1. Whisk the eggs, egg whites and parsley in a bowl until well combined. Season with freshly ground black pepper.

2. Lightly spray a non-stick frying pan with olive oil and heat over medium–low heat. Pour in the egg mixture and cook for 30 seconds or until the mixture starts to set around the edges. Using a wooden spoon, gently stir for 1–2 minutes or until the egg has just set.

3. Meanwhile, place the baby spinach in a small heatproof bowl and cover with boiling water. Set aside for 1 minute to wilt, then drain well.

4. Divide the spinach, scrambled eggs, avocado and tomatoes between two plates. Season with freshly ground black pepper and serve.

286 Calories   3.6 g Carbs

Nutritional Information

(per serve)

Calories	**286**
Protein	**14.4 g**
Fat Total	**23.7 g**
Fat Saturated	**5.5 g**
Carbohydrates	**3.6 g**
Sugars	**2.3 g**
Sodium	**179.6 mg**
Dietary Fibre	**4.3 g**

Mish Tips

Take care not to overcook the scrambled eggs or they will become dry and rubbery.

Thai fish cakes with bean sprout salad

Thai food has always been top of my yum list and this recipe is no exception. These fish cakes are dead easy and so tasty. If you like a little spice, add some chopped fresh chilli.

Serves: **2** · Prep time: **20 minutes, plus 30 minutes chilling** · Cooking time: **10 minutes** · Great for: *Dinner*

Ingredients

500 g white fish fillets, skin and bones removed, roughly chopped

1 tablespoon green curry paste

1 spring onion, finely sliced

½ cup coriander leaves

1 teaspoon olive oil

60 g bean sprouts, trimmed

1 carrot, cut into ribbons

1 Lebanese cucumber, halved lengthways and sliced

2 limes, cut into wedges

Method

1. Place the fish in a food processor and blitz to a coarse paste. Transfer to a bowl and add the curry paste and spring onion. Finely chop half the coriander, add to the fish mixture and stir until well combined.

2. Using clean hands, shape the mixture into six even patties. Place on a plate, cover with plastic film and refrigerate for 30 minutes.

3. Heat the olive oil in a large non-stick frying pan over medium heat. Add the chilled patties and flatten them slightly, then cook for 3–4 minutes each side or until nicely golden and cooked through.

4. Meanwhile, place the bean sprouts, carrot, cucumber and remaining coriander leaves in a bowl and gently toss to combine.

5. Divide the fish cakes and salad between two plates and serve with the lime wedges on the side.

272	4.9 g
Calories	Carbs

Nutritional Information
(per serve)

Calories	**272**
Protein	**41.6 g**
Fat Total	**8.1 g**
Fat Saturated	**1.6 g**
Carbohydrates	**4.9 g**
Sugars	**4.4 g**
Sodium	**211.9 mg**
Dietary Fibre	**5.1 g**

Mish Tips

Use a vegetable peeler to cut the carrot into ribbons.

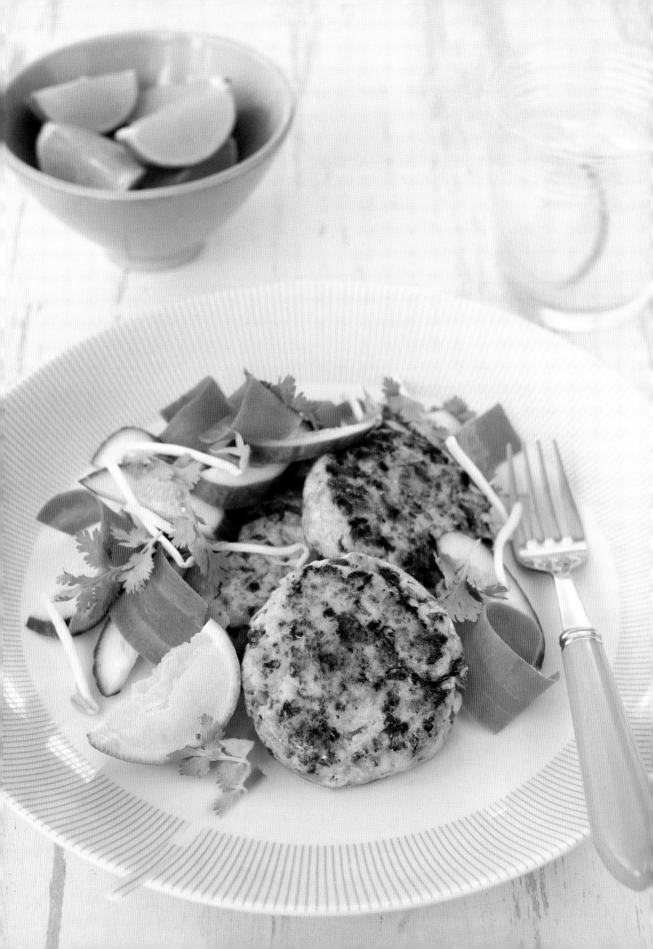

Salmon, avocado and walnut salad

Good fats, good health, good times. Go you!

Serves: **2** · Prep time: **15 minutes** · Cooking time: **10 minutes** · Great for: *Lunch*

Ingredients

180 g Atlantic salmon fillet, skin and
    bones removed

olive oil spray

100 g baby potatoes, quartered

1 celery stalk, finely sliced

1 spring onion, sliced

40 g avocado

30 g baby spinach leaves

5 g walnuts, toasted, roughly chopped

1 tablespoon lemon juice

1 clove garlic, crushed

Method

1. Heat a chargrill pan or non-stick frying pan over medium heat. Lightly spray the salmon with olive oil and season with freshly ground black pepper. Add to the pan and cook for 3 minutes each side or until just cooked through. Transfer to a plate and set aside to cool slightly, then break into bite-sized pieces.

2. Meanwhile, place the potato in a microwave-safe bowl with ⅓ cup water. Cover and microwave on high for 5 minutes or until just tender. Uncover, drain and cool.

3. Combine the celery and spring onion in a large bowl. Scoop spoonfuls of avocado into the bowl and add the spinach, walnuts, salmon pieces and cooled potato. Season with freshly ground black pepper.

4. Whisk together the lemon juice and garlic in a small bowl or jug. Pour over the salad and gently toss to combine, then serve.

288 Calories   **8.2** g Carbs

Nutritional Information

(per serve)

Calories	**288**
Protein	**21.4 g**
Fat Total	**18.7 g**
Fat Saturated	**4.5 g**
Carbohydrates	**8.2 g**
Sugars	**1.4 g**
Sodium	**80.5 mg**
Dietary Fibre	**2.6 g**

Souffle omelette with spinach and mushrooms

Souffle without any stress? Yep, it can be done! The air beaten into the egg whites makes this omelette super light and fluffy. It's so delicious.

Serves: **2** · Prep time: **20 minutes** · Cooking time: **15 minutes** · Great for: *Breakfast*

Ingredients

3 teaspoons olive oil
1 red onion, finely sliced
100 g mushrooms, sliced
1 clove garlic, crushed
150 g English spinach, trimmed and roughly chopped
55 g drained and rinsed tinned lentils
3 cage-free eggs
3 cage-free egg whites
olive oil spray
30 g goat's cheese

Method

1. Heat the olive oil in a non-stick frying pan over medium heat. Add the onion and cook for 3 minutes or until softened. Add the mushroom and cook for a further 3–4 minutes or until browned. Add the garlic and spinach and toss until the spinach has wilted. Stir in the lentils, then set aside, covered to keep warm.

2. Meanwhile, whisk the eggs in a large bowl. Place the egg whites in a separate clean bowl and beat with electric beaters until soft peaks form. Working in three batches, carefully fold the egg whites through the whisked eggs using a large metal spoon.

3. Preheat the grill to medium–high. Lightly spray a small non-stick frying pan with olive oil and heat over medium heat. Spoon half the egg mixture into the pan, spreading it out to the edge, and cook for 1–2 minutes or until set underneath. Place under the grill and cook for a further 1–2 minutes or until puffed and golden.

4. Transfer to a serving plate. Spoon half the spinach mixture onto one half of the omelette and crumble over half the goat's cheese. Fold the omelette over to cover the filling. Serve. Repeat with the remaining ingredients to make the second omelette; or have two pans on the go at once.

314	5.8 g
Calories	Carbs

Nutritional Information
(per serve)

Calories	**314**
Protein	**25.6 g**
Fat Total	**20.4 g**
Fat Saturated	**5.7 g**
Carbohydrates	**5.8 g**
Sugars	**3.6 g**
Sodium	**355.9 mg**
Dietary Fibre	**5.1 g**

Mish Tips

This recipe is delicious using Swiss brown or fresh shiitake mushrooms. If your frying pan doesn't have a heatproof handle, wrap it in a damp tea towel to protect it under the grill. Take care as the tea towel will get hot.

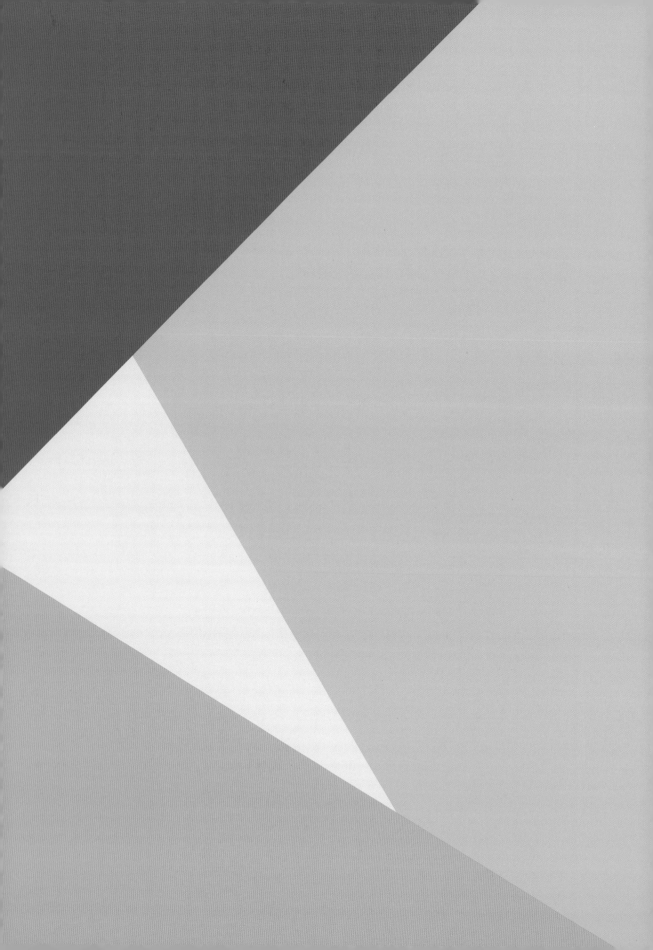

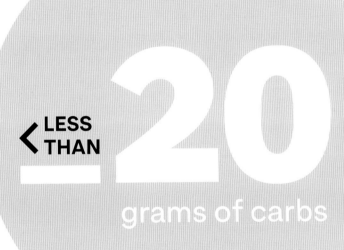

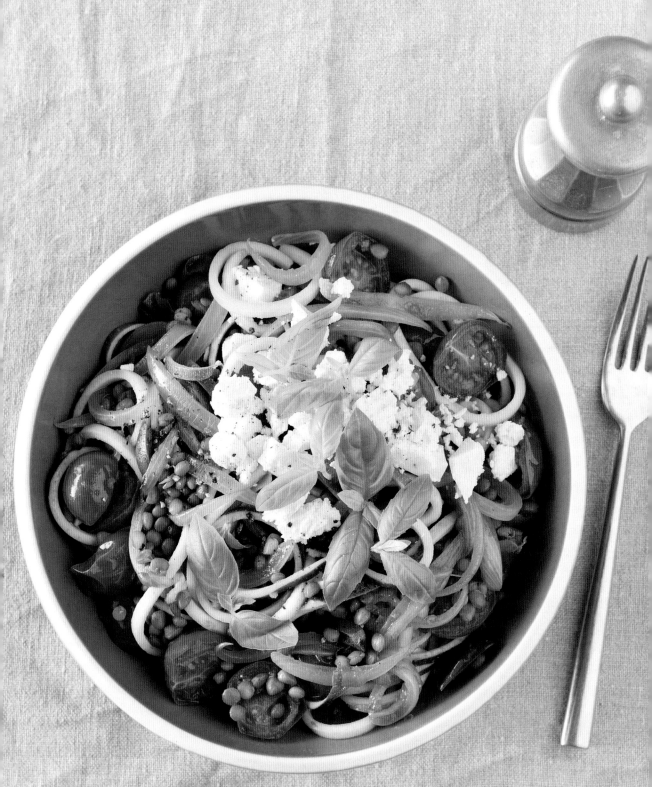

Zucchini noodles with lentils and feta

Zoodles are all the rage these days and with good reason — all the fun of a bowl of pasta without the carb overload. This vego version uses lentils and feta for protein. Win—win!

Serves: **2** • Prep time: **10 minutes** • Cooking time: **10 minutes** • Great for: *Lunch, Dinner or Leftovers*

299	17 g
Calories	Carbs

Ingredients

2 teaspoons olive oil

3 zucchini, cut into noodles

½ brown onion, finely sliced

1 clove garlic, crushed

250 g cherry tomatoes, halved

1 x 400 g tin lentils, drained and rinsed

10 kalamata olives, pitted and halved

2 tablespoons lemon juice

80 g low-fat feta, crumbled

3 tablespoons basil leaves

Method

1. Heat half the olive oil in a large deep non-stick frying pan over medium heat. Add the zucchini noodles and cook, tossing regularly, for 2 minutes or until just softened. Transfer to a large bowl.

2. Heat the remaining oil in the pan. Add the onion and cook, stirring occasionally, for 3 minutes or until softened. Add the garlic and tomatoes and cook, tossing and stirring, for 2 minutes or until the tomatoes have softened. Stir in the lentils, olives and lemon juice until heated through.

3. Divide the zucchini noodles between two bowls and top with the lentil mixture. Scatter over the feta and basil, season with freshly ground black pepper and serve.

Nutritional Information

(per serve)

Calories	**299**
Protein	**19.2 g**
Fat Total	**15.0 g**
Fat Saturated	**8.7 g**
Carbohydrates	**17.0 g**
Sugars	**8.3 g**
Sodium	**1021.0 mg**
Dietary Fibre	**5.7 g**

Mish Tips

Use a spiraliser or julienne peeler to cut the zucchini into noodles. Alternatively, just cut them into very thin slices.

Grated beetroot and chickpea fritters

These gluten-free fritters look like they sprang from the coolest cafe — at a fraction of the price, I'm sure!

Serves: **2** · Prep time: **20 minutes** · Cooking time: **10 minutes** · Great for: *Breakfast or Lunch*

Ingredients

1 x 400 g tin chickpeas, drained and rinsed

2 cage-free eggs, lightly beaten

50 g beetroot, grated

1 spring onion, chopped

1½ teaspoons Moroccan seasoning

olive oil spray

30 g mixed salad leaves

½ Lebanese cucumber, halved lengthways and sliced

2 tablespoons low-fat cottage cheese

¼ avocado, diced

Method

1. Coarsely mash the chickpeas in a large bowl, then add the egg, beetroot, spring onion and Moroccan seasoning and stir until just combined.

2. Lightly spray a large non-stick frying pan with olive oil and heat over medium heat. Divide the mixture into four equal portions, then drop into the pan and spread out until 9 cm in diameter. Cook for 3–4 minutes each side or until cooked through and lightly golden.

3. Divide the salad leaves and cucumber between two bowls and add the fritters. Top with the cottage cheese and avocado, season with freshly ground black pepper and serve.

291	**18.9** g
Calories	Carbs

Nutritional Information
(per serve)

Calories	**291**
Protein	**18.9 g**
Fat Total	**14.5 g**
Fat Saturated	**3.6 g**
Carbohydrates	**18.9 g**
Sugars	**4.2 g**
Sodium	**463.7 mg**
Dietary Fibre	**7.4 g**

Mish Tips

Moroccan seasoning is a spice blend comprising ginger, white pepper, coriander, turmeric, allspice, and cinnamon. If you have these ingredients at home, you could make up some of your own. For convenience, I usually use a ready-made one.

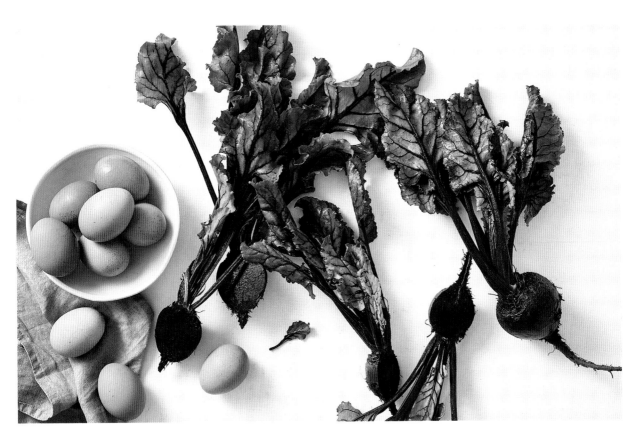

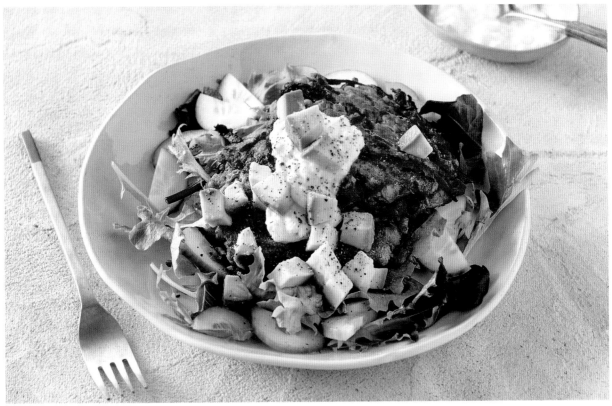

Less than 20 grams of carbs

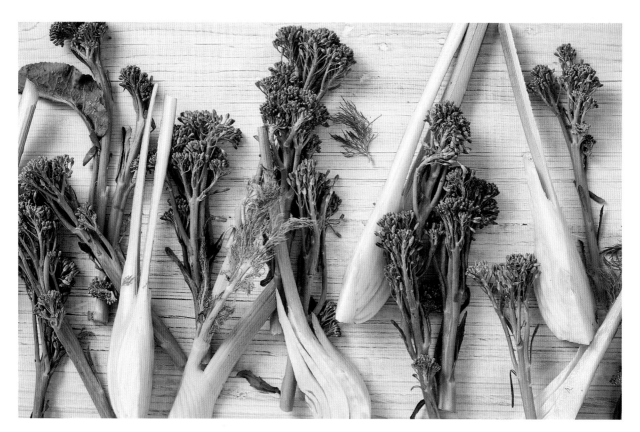

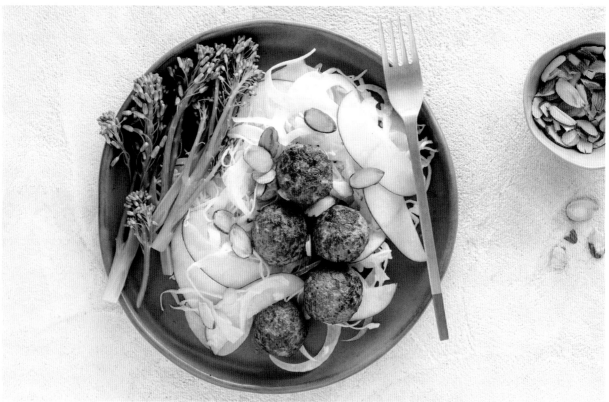

Pork meatballs with fennel and apple slaw

Enjoy these tasty meatballs without heavy carb-laden pasta, and go for a zingy slaw instead.

Serves: **2** • Prep time: **25 minutes** • Cooking time: **10 minutes** • Great for: *Lunch or Leftovers*

311 **Calories**   13.4 g **Carbs**

Ingredients

200 g lean pork mince

1 teaspoon finely grated ginger

1 clove garlic, crushed

½ teaspoon chilli paste

olive oil spray

1 bunch broccolini, trimmed

1 red apple, quartered, cored and finely sliced

1 baby fennel bulb, trimmed, halved and finely sliced

60 g white cabbage, shredded

2 spring onions, finely sliced

1½ tablespoons low-fat natural yoghurt

2 tablespoons lemon juice

10 g flaked almonds, toasted

Method

1. Mix together the pork mince, ginger, garlic and chilli paste until well combined. Roll level tablespoons of the mixture into balls (you should get 10). Heat a non-stick frying pan over medium heat. Lightly spray the meatballs with olive oil and cook for 10 minutes, shaking the pan and turning occasionally to brown evenly.

2. Meanwhile, steam the broccolini for about 3 minutes or until tender.

3. Combine the apple, fennel, cabbage and spring onion in a large bowl and toss with the yoghurt and lemon juice. Season with freshly ground black pepper.

4. Serve the meatballs with the broccolini and slaw. Finish with a sprinkling of flaked almonds.

Nutritional Information

(per serve)

Calories	**311**
Protein	**27.0 g**
Fat Total	**15.1 g**
Fat Saturated	**4.2 g**
Carbohydrates	**13.4 g**
Sugars	**12.9 g**
Sodium	**138.2 mg**
Dietary Fibre	**7.3 g**

Mish Tips

Pork is one of the leanest proteins around, so you can enjoy it knowing that you're getting lots of valuable protein to fuel your body.

Warm *Mediterranean* beef salad

You won't miss carbs with this satisfying warm salad, full of hearty Mediterranean flavours.

Serves: **2** • Prep time: **10 minutes** • Cooking time: **30 minutes** • Great for: *Weekend Lunch or Dinner*

Ingredients

1 red onion, cut into wedges
2 zucchini, sliced
200 g cherry tomatoes, halved
100 g red capsicum, seeded and sliced
finely grated zest of 1 lemon
1 clove garlic, crushed
2 tablespoons chopped oregano, plus
   extra leaves to serve
olive oil spray
200 g lean rump steak
50 g low-fat feta, crumbled

Method

1. Preheat the oven to 200°C (180°C fan-forced). Line a large baking tray with baking paper.

2. Place the onion, zucchini, tomatoes and capsicum in a large bowl. Gently toss through the lemon zest, garlic and chopped oregano, and season with freshly ground black pepper.

3. Spread the vegetables over the prepared tray and lightly spray with olive oil. Bake for 30 minutes or until lightly golden and tender.

4. Meanwhile, heat a non-stick frying pan over medium heat. Season the beef with freshly ground black pepper and lightly spray with olive oil. Cook for 2–3 minutes each side for medium–rare, or until cooked to your liking. Transfer to a plate, cover with foil and leave to rest for 5 minutes.

5. Divide the vegetables between two plates. Slice the beef and add to plates, top with the feta, then sprinkle with the extra oregano and serve.

304	11.7 g
Calories	Carbs

Nutritional Information
(per serve)

Calories	**304**
Protein	**30.6 g**
Fat Total	**12.9 g**
Fat Saturated	**6.8 g**
Carbohydrates	**11.7 g**
Sugars	**8.0 g**
Sodium	**542.8 mg**
Dietary Fibre	**11.1 g**

Mish Tips

To add extra flavour, chargrill the capsicum before baking with the other vegetables. To do this, cut it into large pieces and remove the seeds and membrane. Place, skin side up, under a hot grill or, skin side down, on a hot chargrill pan and cook until the skin has blistered and blackened. Let it cool, then remove the skin and cut the flesh as required. Alternatively, buy it in jars from the supermarket or your local deli.

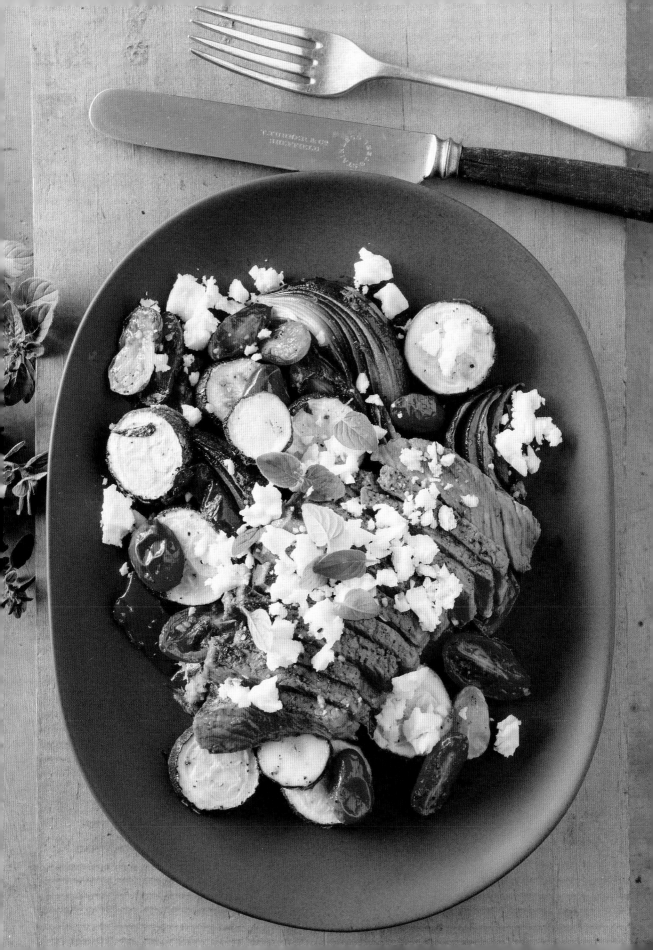

Ginger and lemongrass roast chicken

A fabulous low-carb roast with an Asian twist!

Serves: **4** · Prep time: **15 minutes** · Cooking time: **40 minutes** · Great for: *Lunch, Dinner or Leftovers*

Ingredients

1 lemongrass stalk, white part only, finely chopped
2 teaspoons chilli paste
3 teaspoons finely grated ginger
1 clove garlic, crushed
1 tablespoon olive oil
500 g lean chicken breast fillets
2 zucchini, sliced
2 carrots, sliced
300 g cauliflower, cut into florets
1 x 400 g tin chickpeas, drained and rinsed
2 teaspoons sesame seeds, toasted
80 g mixed salad leaves

Method

1. Preheat the oven to 190°C (170°C fan-forced). Line a large baking tray with baking paper.

2. Combine the lemongrass, chilli paste, ginger, garlic and 1 teaspoon olive oil in a small bowl. Place the chicken on the prepared tray and evenly spread with the paste mix.

3. Toss the zucchini, carrot, cauliflower and chickpeas with the remaining oil, and arrange around the chicken. Season with freshly ground black pepper. Roast for 30–40 minutes or until the chicken is cooked through and the vegetables are tender and lightly golden.

4. Thickly slice the chicken. Divide the chicken and vegetables among plates and sprinkle with the sesame seeds. Serve with the salad leaves on the side.

287	12.3 g
Calories	Carbs

Nutritional Information

(per serve)

Calories	**287**
Protein	**34.4 g**
Fat Total	**9.7 g**
Fat Saturated	**1.6 g**
Carbohydrates	**12.3 g**
Sugars	**4.6 g**
Sodium	**277.6 mg**
Dietary Fibre	**7.2 g**

Mish Tips

If you like, replace the fresh lemongrass with 1 tablespoon lemongrass paste (available near the fresh herbs at the supermarket).

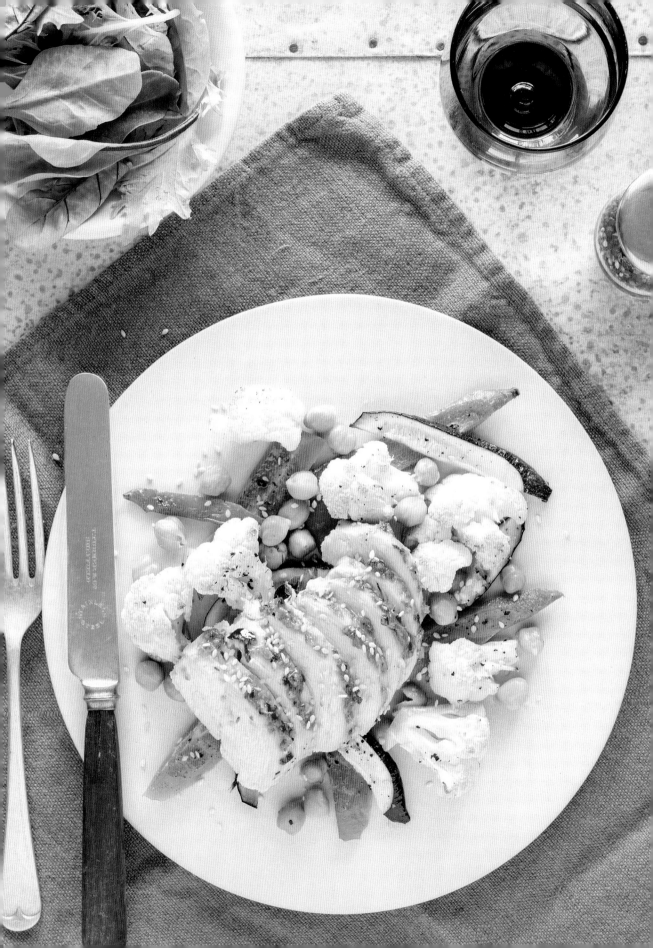

Mild chicken *korma*

While still full of flavour, this curry isn't too spicy at all – just a warming bowl of comfort the whole family will love. Freeze ahead for easy meal planning.

Serves: **6** • Prep time: **15 minutes** • Cooking time: **30 minutes** • Great for: *Lunch, Dinner or Leftovers*

291	19 g
Calories	Carbs

Ingredients

1 tablespoon olive oil

600 g lean chicken thigh fillets, chopped

1 brown onion, halved and sliced

3 tablespoons korma curry paste

1 x 400 g tin diced tomatoes

1 cup salt-reduced chicken stock

1 x 270 ml tin low-fat coconut milk

500 g sweet potato, peeled and chopped

200 g green beans, trimmed and halved

3 tablespoons chopped coriander

Method

1. Heat half the olive oil in a large non-stick saucepan over medium–high heat. Add the chicken in two batches and cook for about 3 minutes each, turning to brown evenly. Transfer to a plate and set aside.

2. Reduce the heat to medium and heat the remaining oil in the pan. Add the onion and cook, stirring occasionally, for 5 minutes or until golden brown. Stir in the curry paste and cook for 1 minute.

3. Add the tomatoes, stock, coconut milk, sweet potato and beans, and return the chicken to the pan. Cover and bring to a simmer, then reduce the heat to low and cook for 10 minutes. Remove the lid and cook for a further 5 minutes or until the sauce has thickened slightly.

4. Spoon the curry into bowls, sprinkle with the coriander and serve.

Nutritional Information
(per serve)

Calories	**291**
Protein	**22.8 g**
Fat Total	**12.9 g**
Fat Saturated	**5.2 g**
Carbohydrates	**19.0 g**
Sugars	**10.3 g**
Sodium	**428.4 mg**
Dietary Fibre	**5.0 g**

Mish Tips

If you are cooking ahead for quick weeknight meals, cool the curry completely, then divide into serving portions and freeze in an airtight container for up to 2 months.

Chicken, pumpkin and chickpeas

Don't you love a 'one pot' meal? Less washing up means more time to do fun stuff!

Serves: **4** · Prep time: **10 minutes** · Cooking time: **35 minutes** · Great for: *Dinner*

Ingredients

1 teaspoon olive oil

500 g lean chicken thigh fillets, chopped

1 red onion, sliced

400 g peeled pumpkin, diced

2 cloves garlic, crushed

¼ teaspoon ground cinnamon

½ cup salt-reduced chicken stock

1 x 400 g tin chickpeas, drained and rinsed

100 g baby spinach leaves

1 spring onion, finely chopped

Method

1. Heat the olive oil in a large non-stick frying pan over medium–high heat. Add the chicken in two batches and cook for about 5 minutes each, turning occasionally until golden. Transfer to a plate and set aside.

2. Reheat the pan. Add the onion and cook, stirring, for 3 minutes or until just softened. Add the pumpkin and cook, turning occasionally, for 7 minutes or until the edges begin to caramelise. Stir in the garlic and cinnamon.

3. Add the stock and chickpeas, and return the chicken to the pan. Cover and simmer for 3 minutes, then remove the lid and simmer for a further 5–10 minutes or until the liquid has reduced and the pumpkin is tender. Stir through the spinach and spring onion and allow to wilt. Season with freshly ground black pepper and serve.

285 Calories   **17.5 g** Carbs

Nutritional Information
(per serve)

Calories	**285**
Protein	**29.5 g**
Fat Total	**9.1 g**
Fat Saturated	**2.2 g**
Carbohydrates	**17.5 g**
Sugars	**8.8 g**
Sodium	**322.5 mg**
Dietary Fibre	**7.0 g**

Mish Tips

Replace the baby spinach with baby kale leaves (available at your supermarket).

Lentil salad with poached eggs

Lentils and eggs are great sources of protein for vegetarians, and here you get both in one delicious salad.

Serves: **2** • Prep time: **10 minutes** • Cooking time: **5 minutes** • Great for: *Breakfast or Lunch*

Ingredients

1 x 400 g tin lentils, drained and rinsed

½ red onion, finely sliced

60 g mixed salad leaves

1½ tablespoons currants

2 cage-free eggs

40 g low-fat feta, crumbled

2 teaspoons olive oil

2 teaspoons dukkah

Method

1. Divide the lentils, onion, salad leaves and currants between two bowls. Season with freshly ground black pepper and set aside.

2. Bring a medium saucepan of water to a simmer. Crack one egg into a small bowl. Stir the water to create a whirlpool, then gently slide the egg into the water. Repeat with the second egg, then simmer for 2 minutes for a soft yolk, or until cooked to your liking. Lift the eggs out with a slotted spoon and place one on each bowl.

3. Top with the feta and a drizzle of olive oil, then sprinkle with the dukkah and serve.

297	16.9 g
Calories	Carbs

Nutritional Information

(per serve)

Calories	**297**
Protein	**20.2 g**
Fat Total	**15.7 g**
Fat Saturated	**6.2 g**
Carbohydrates	**16.9 g**
Sugars	**8.6 g**
Sodium	**655.3 mg**
Dietary Fibre	**2.2 g**

Mish Tips

Dukkah is an Egyptian spice mix of dried herbs, sesame seeds, nuts and spices. Look for it in the spice section of your supermarket. If you can't find it, use a blend of equal parts sesame seeds and ground cumin.

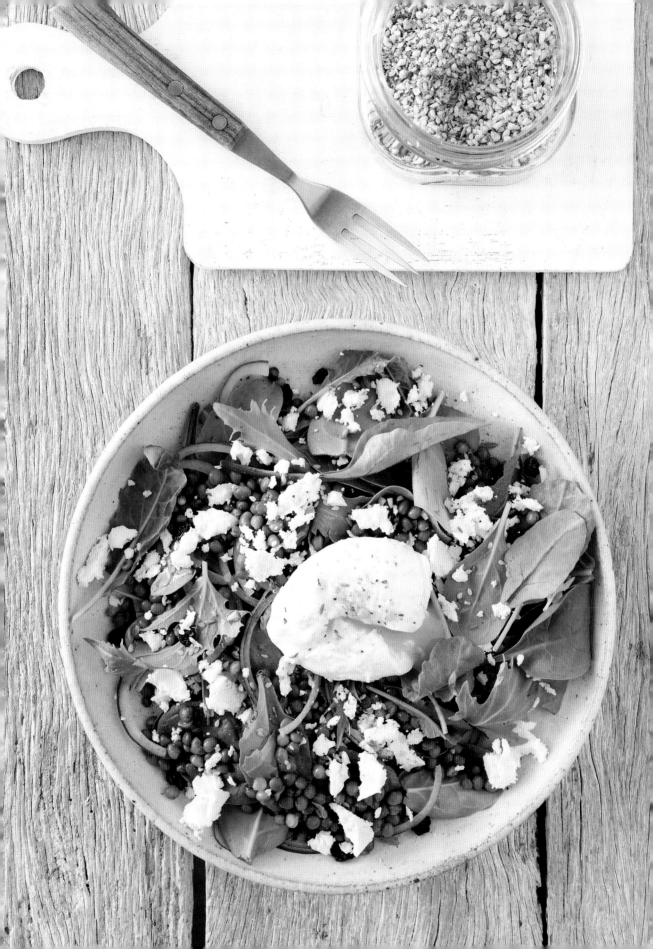

Chicken and lettuce 'tacos'

Tacos are very popular in our household, and this is a fantastic low-carb way to enjoy a Mexican meal.

Serves: **2** • Prep time: **10 minutes** • Cooking time: **10 minutes** • Great for: *Weekend Lunch or Dinner*

326 Calories 17.2 g Carbs

Ingredients

200 g lean chicken thigh fillets

finely grated zest and juice of 1 lime

¼ teaspoon chilli powder

olive oil spray

2 tomatoes, chopped

2 spring onions, sliced

1 x 125 g tin corn kernels, drained

6 cos lettuce leaves

1 red capsicum, seeded and cut into thin strips

1 tablespoon extra light sour cream

50 g low-fat cheddar, grated

Method

1. Preheat a barbecue grill to medium–high or heat a chargrill pan over medium–high heat. Cut deep slashes into the chicken. Combine the lime zest and juice and chilli powder and rub all over the chicken. Lightly spray with olive oil, and cook, turning once, for 6 minutes or until golden brown and cooked through. Cool slightly, then cut into thin strips.

2. Combine the tomato, spring onion and corn in a bowl.

3. Divide the tomato mixture among the lettuce leaves and drizzle with a little sour cream. Top with the capsicum and chicken, sprinkle with the cheese and serve.

Nutritional Information
(per serve)

Calories	**326**
Protein	**31.4 g**
Fat Total	**13.9 g**
Fat Saturated	**6.4 g**
Carbohydrates	**17.2 g**
Sugars	**10.2 g**
Sodium	**368.9 mg**
Dietary Fibre	**6.6 g**

Mish Tips

Use small or baby cos lettuce for this recipe.

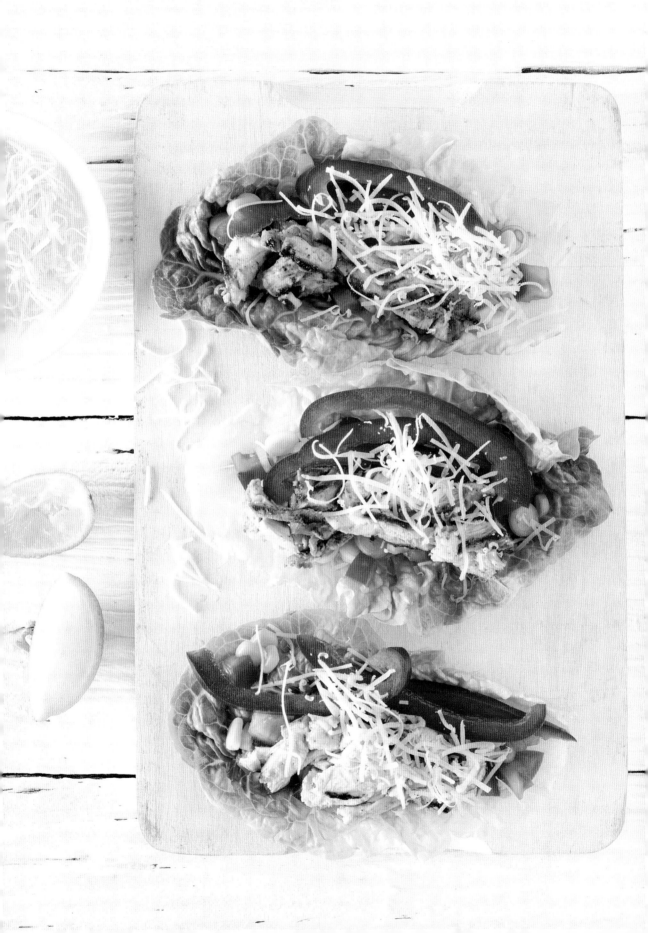

Lamb slaw

Power up with this protein-packed slaw. Yummo!

Serves: **2** · Prep time: **10 minutes** · Cooking time: **10 minutes** · Great for: *Lunch*

321 Calories   13 g Carbs

Ingredients

1 teaspoon Greek seasoning
250 g lamb loin fillet
olive oil spray
1 red apple, quartered, cored and
    finely sliced
½ cup mint leaves
200 g white cabbage, shredded
1 tablespoon sunflower seeds
juice of ½ lemon

Method

1. Heat a non-stick frying pan over medium-high heat. Sprinkle the Greek seasoning over the lamb and lightly spray with olive oil. Cook the lamb for 3 minutes each side for medium–rare, or until cooked to your liking. Transfer to a plate, cover loosely with foil and rest for a few minutes before slicing.

2. Combine the apple, mint, cabbage and sunflower seeds in a large bowl. Finely slice the lamb and add to the slaw, then squeeze over the lemon juice. Season with freshly ground black pepper and toss to combine. Divide between bowls and serve.

Nutritional Information
(per serve)

Calories	**321**
Protein	**39.9 g**
Fat Total	**10.7 g**
Fat Saturated	**2.7 g**
Carbohydrates	**13.0 g**
Sugars	**12.2 g**
Sodium	**225.5 mg**
Dietary Fibre	**6.1 g**

As pictured, try using kale slaw in place of the cabbage mixture. This packaged mixture of shredded carrot, beetroot, cabbage and kale is available in the fresh fruit and veggie section at the supermarket.

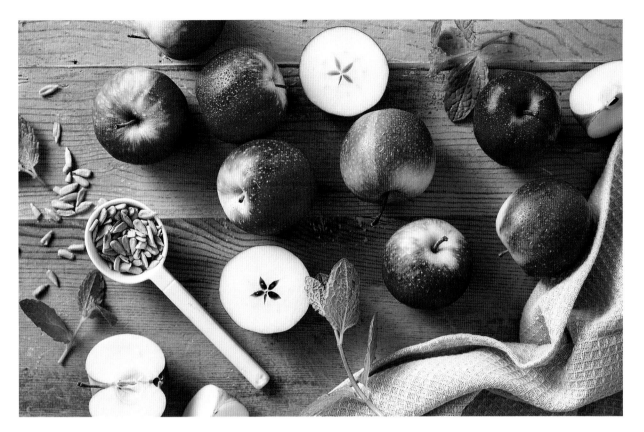

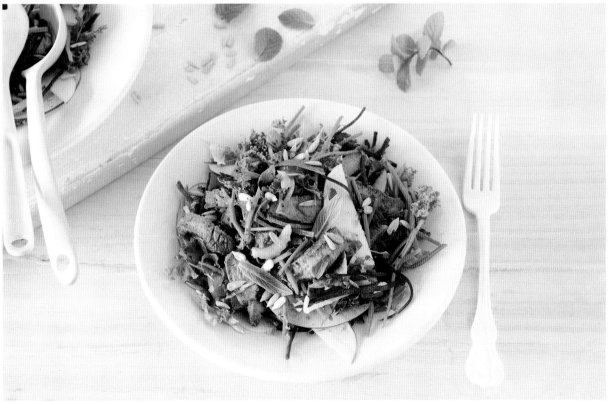

Baked mushrooms

We all know mushrooms are delicious, but they are also super filling and packed full of protein, so this recipe really hits the spot on all fronts!

Serves: **2** • Prep time: **15 minutes** • Cooking time: **25 minutes** • Great for: *Weekend Breakfast*

290	14.1 g
Calories	Carbs

Ingredients

4 large mushrooms, stems removed and finely chopped

1 zucchini, grated and squeezed to remove excess moisture

2 spring onions, chopped

2 cloves garlic, finely chopped

finely grated zest and juice of 1 lemon

180 g lean beef mince

⅓ cup puffed rice

1 tablespoon chopped dill

olive oil spray

35 g low-fat feta

Method

1. Preheat the oven to 200°C (180°C fan-forced). Line a baking tray with baking paper. Place the mushroom cups, stem side up, on the tray.

2. Place the chopped mushroom stalk, zucchini, spring onion, garlic, lemon zest, beef mince, puffed rice and dill in a large bowl. Season with freshly ground black pepper and mix until well combined.

3. Stuff each mushroom cup with the filling, piling it high. Lightly spray with olive oil and bake for 20–25 minutes or until the filling is cooked and golden and the mushrooms are tender. Crumble the feta over the top and squeeze over a little lemon juice, then serve immediately.

Nutritional Information
(per serve)

Calories	**290**
Protein	**36.0 g**
Fat Total	**10.0 g**
Fat Saturated	**6.4 g**
Carbohydrates	**14.1 g**
Sugars	**5.2 g**
Sodium	**279.7 mg**
Dietary Fibre	**6.2 g**

We used portobello mushrooms (the lovely brown ones) in this recipe, but you can use large cap or field mushrooms if preferred. You want each mushroom to weigh about 70 g.

Barbecued steak with iceberg lettuce

This super simple, mid-week dinner is very popular in our house. I sometimes rub the spice mix over the corn too. It's absolutely delicious cooked on the barbecue!

Serves: **2** · Prep time: **15 minutes, plus 10 minutes standing** · Cooking time: **5 minutes** ·
Great for: *Weekend Lunch or Dinner*

276 · Calories
12.5 g · Carbs

Ingredients

1 teaspoon brown sugar
1 teaspoon ground cumin
½ teaspoon sweet paprika
½ teaspoon cayenne pepper
2 x 125 g lean beef fillets, fat trimmed
1 corn cob, husk and silks removed, halved
olive oil spray
60 g iceberg lettuce leaves
1 Lebanese cucumber, chopped
1 lime, cut into wedges

Method

1. Combine the sugar, cumin, paprika and cayenne pepper in a small bowl. Put the steak in a shallow dish and sprinkle the spice mix over both sides. Set aside for 10 minutes.

2. Place the corn in a shallow microwave safe-dish and add 3 tablespoons water. Cover and microwave on high for 4 minutes or until tender.

3. Meanwhile, heat a chargrill pan over medium–high heat. Lightly spray both sides of the steak with olive oil, then cook for 2 minutes each side for medium, or until cooked to your liking. Transfer to a plate to rest for 2 minutes.

4. Divide the steak, corn, iceberg lettuce and cucumber between two plates. Serve with lime wedges on the side.

Nutritional Information
(per serve)

Calories	**276**
Protein	**31.1 g**
Fat Total	**10.1 g**
Fat Saturated	**3.3 g**
Carbohydrates	**12.5 g**
Sugars	**6.3 g**
Sodium	**93.3 mg**
Dietary Fibre	**6 g**

If you don't have any cayenne pepper, just use a pinch of ground chilli instead. You can also replace the sweet paprika with smoked paprika.

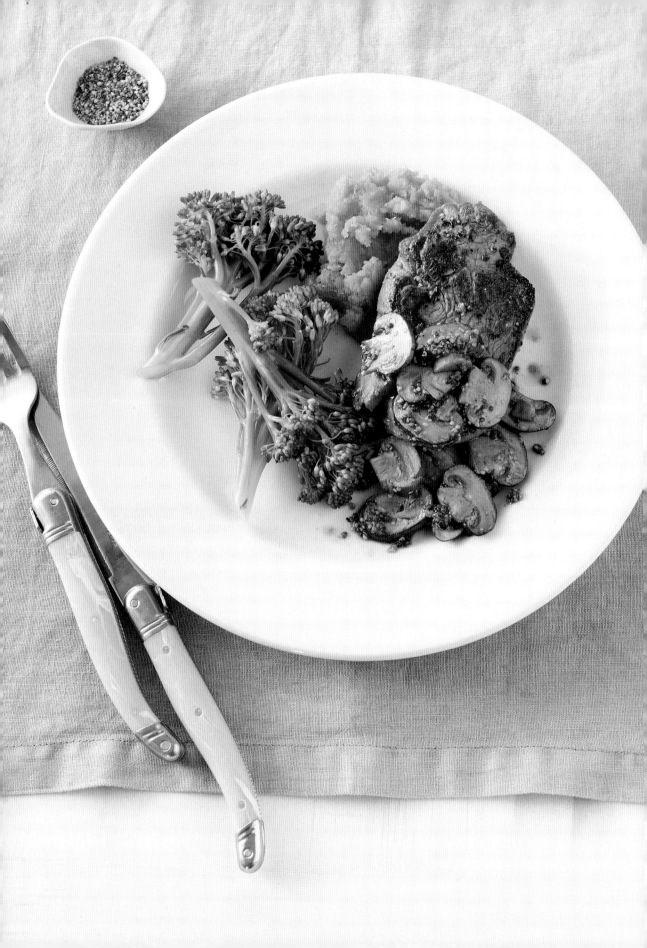

Beef and mushrooms with mash

Cannellini beans and wholegrain mustard give this hearty meal a delicious depth of flavour that the whole family will enjoy.

Serves: **2** · Prep time: **10 minutes** · Cooking time: **10 minutes** · Great for: *Dinner*

Ingredients

150 g sweet potato, peeled and chopped

100 g drained and rinsed tinned cannellini beans

2 x 100 g blade steaks

olive oil spray

100 g mushrooms, sliced

1 clove garlic, crushed

1 teaspoon wholegrain mustard

100 g broccolini, trimmed

Method

1. Place the sweet potato in a microwave-safe bowl and add 3 tablespoons water. Cover and microwave on high for 5 minutes or until soft. Drain. Add the cannellini beans and mash well.

2. While the sweet potato is cooking, heat a non-stick frying pan over medium–high heat. Lightly spray the steaks with olive oil and season with freshly ground black pepper. Cook for 2 minutes each side for medium–rare, or until cooked to your liking. Transfer to a plate, cover loosely with foil and set aside to rest.

3. Add the mushroom to the pan and cook, stirring, for 2 minutes. Add the garlic and mustard and cook, stirring, for 2 minutes or until the mushroom is lightly golden. Add a splash of water if the mixture is a little dry.

4. Meanwhile, steam the broccolini in the microwave for 3–4 minutes or until just tender.

5. Serve the steaks with the mash, mushroom and broccolini.

304 Calories   **17.7** g Carbs

Nutritional Information

(per serve)

Calories	**304**
Protein	**29.7 g**
Fat Total	**11.0 g**
Fat Saturated	**3.8 g**
Carbohydrates	**17.7 g**
Sugars	**5.7 g**
Sodium	**271.7 mg**
Dietary Fibre	**8.3 g**

Mish Tips

Buy pre-sliced mushrooms to save time.

Turkey meatballs in tomato sauce

Turkey is a great lean protein that works wonderfully well here.
The meatballs are full of flavour without the fat.

Serves: **2** · Prep time: **20 minutes** · Cooking time: **30 minutes** · Great for: *Lunch, Dinner or Leftovers*

Ingredients

250 g turkey mince

2 tablespoons quinoa, rinsed
  and drained

½ teaspoon vegetable stock powder

2 teaspoons olive oil

1 carrot, grated

1 red capsicum, seeded and
  finely chopped

1 zucchini, chopped

2 cloves garlic, crushed

200 g tinned diced tomatoes

30 g baby rocket leaves

Method

1. Combine the mince, quinoa and stock powder in a bowl and season with freshly ground black pepper. Roll the mixture into walnut-sized balls.

2. Heat the olive oil in a non-stick frying pan over medium–low heat. Add the meatballs and cook, turning often, for 3 minutes or until lightly browned. Transfer to a plate and set aside.

3. Add the carrot, capsicum and zucchini to the pan and cook, stirring, for 5 minutes or until softened. Add the garlic and cook for 1 minute. Stir in the tomatoes and ¾ cup water and simmer, covered, for 5 minutes.

4. Return the meatballs to the pan and turn to coat in the sauce. Reduce the heat to low and simmer, covered, for 15 minutes or until cooked through and the sauce has thickened slightly. Season with freshly ground black pepper and serve with the rocket leaves.

317 Calories   19.5 g Carbs

Nutritional Information
(per serve)

Calories	**317**
Protein	**32.4 g**
Fat Total	**10.8 g**
Fat Saturated	**2.0 g**
Carbohydrates	**19.5 g**
Sugars	**8.4 g**
Sodium	**574.1 mg**
Dietary Fibre	**6.0 g**

Mish Tips

If you can't find turkey mince, use chicken mince or even lean beef mince.

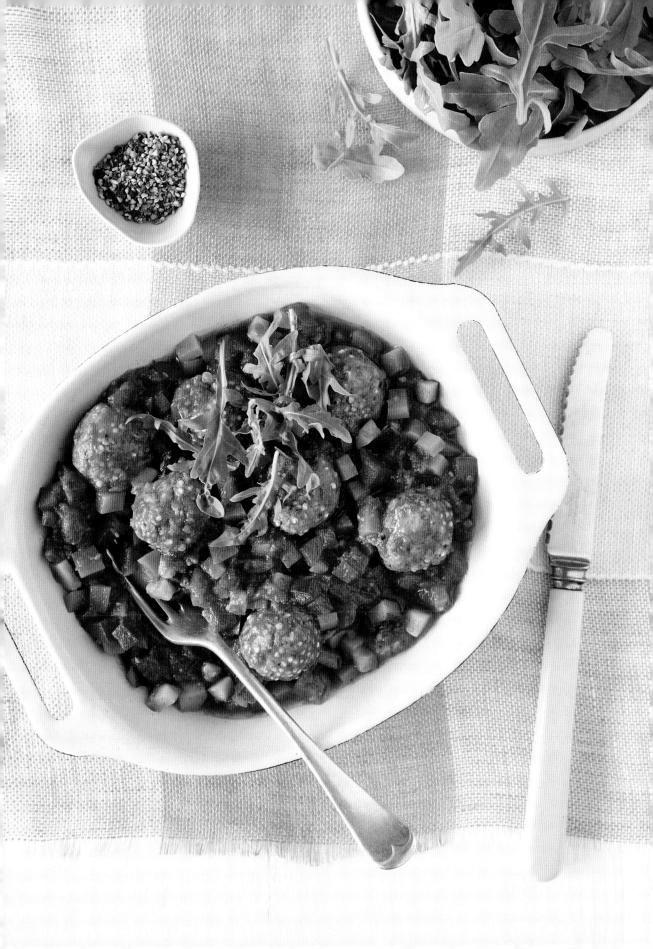

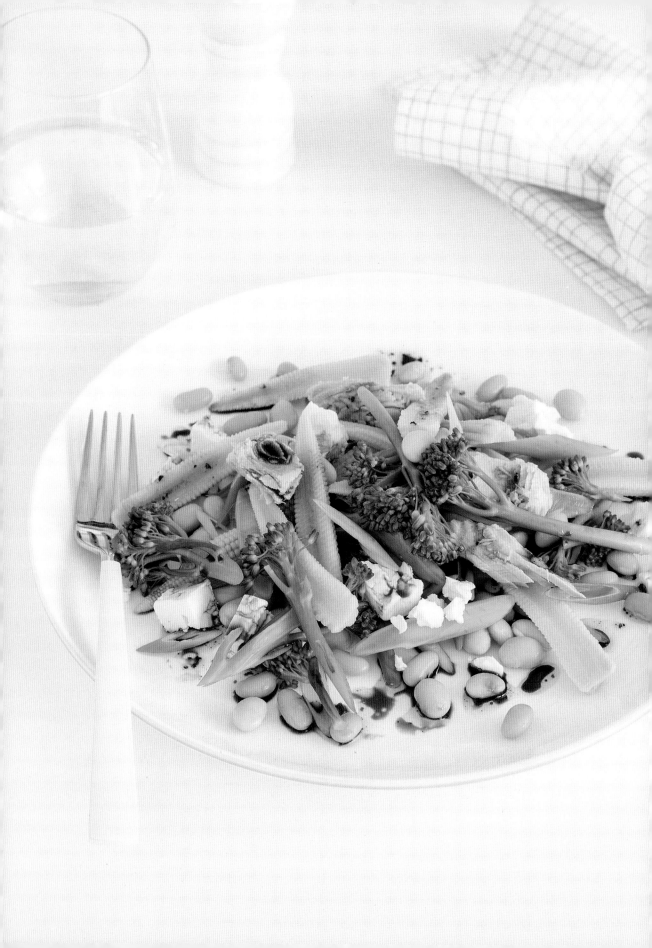

Salmon and edamame salad

This super quick dish uses pantry staples tinned salmon and cannellini beans. So handy if you have leftovers to use up.

Serves: **2** · Prep time: **15 minutes** · Cooking time: **5 minutes** · Great for: *Lunch, Dinner or Leftovers*

271	12.4 g
Calories	Carbs

Ingredients

80 g thawed, peeled edamame

1 bunch broccolini, trimmed
    and chopped

boiling water, for blanching

115 g baby corn spears, halved
    lengthways

100 g drained and rinsed tinned
    cannellini beans

125 g tinned salmon in spring water,
    drained and flaked

2 spring onions, chopped

20 g low-fat feta, crumbled

1 teaspoon balsamic vinegar

1 teaspoon olive oil

Method

1. Place the edamame and broccolini in a heatproof bowl. Cover with boiling water and set aside for 2 minutes. Drain and rinse under cold water.

2. Combine the corn, cannellini beans, salmon, spring onion, feta, edamame and broccolini in a large bowl. Drizzle over the vinegar and olive oil and toss to combine. Season with freshly ground black pepper and serve.

Nutritional Information

(per serve)

Calories	**271**
Protein	**28.9 g**
Fat Total	**12.4 g**
Fat Saturated	**3.9 g**
Carbohydrates	**12.4 g**
Sugars	**2.4 g**
Sodium	**316.4 mg**
Dietary Fibre	**9.3 g**

Mish Tips

If you're making this ahead to take for lunch, pack it into airtight containers and keep chilled. Pack your dressing separately in a leak-proof container. Edamame are fresh soy beans, available from the freezer section of supermarkets and Asian supermarkets. The weight given here is for peeled beans. If you can only buy them in their pods, you will need to double the weight to yield the required quantity of beans.

Less than 20 grams of carbs

Warm potato salad with prawns and asparagus

Prawns are one of my favourite forms of protein and they really shine in this delicious warm salad.

Serves: **2** · Prep time: **10 minutes** · Cooking time: **10 minutes** · Great for: *Dinner*

Ingredients

200 g small coliban potatoes, quartered

2 teaspoons olive oil

2 cloves garlic, crushed

250 g peeled cooked king prawns

1 bunch asparagus, trimmed and chopped

½ cup frozen peas

finely grated zest and juice of 1 lime

½ cup mint leaves

25 g low-fat feta, crumbled

Method

1. Cook the potato in a saucepan of boiling water for 7 minutes or until just tender.

2. Meanwhile, heat the olive oil in a wok or large non-stick frying pan over medium–high heat. Add the garlic and prawns and stir-fry for 1 minute. Add the asparagus and peas and stir-fry for 2 minutes. Stir in the lime zest and juice.

3. Drain the potato, then toss through the prawn mixture. Add the mint and season with freshly ground black pepper, and toss again. Divide between two bowls, top with the feta and serve.

315	16.6 g
Calories	Carbs

Nutritional Information
(per serve)

Calories	**315**
Protein	**38.9 g**
Fat Total	**8.4 g**
Fat Saturated	**3.4 g**
Carbohydrates	**16.6 g**
Sugars	**2.6 g**
Sodium	**835.0 mg**
Dietary Fibre	**7.1 g**

Mish Tips

You can cook the potato in the microwave if you prefer.

Salmon nicoise salad

This is one of my favourite salads. Packed with protein and flavour, it's absolutely yummo!

Serves: **2** • Prep time: **30 minutes** • Cooking time: **15 minutes** • Great for: *Weekend Lunch or Dinner*

Ingredients

100 g baby potatoes

50 g green beans, trimmed

2 cage-free eggs

130 g drained and flaked tinned salmon
    in spring water

250 g cherry tomatoes, halved

½ cos lettuce, leaves torn

1 tablespoon red wine vinegar

1 teaspoon olive oil

2 teaspoons dijon mustard

1 clove garlic, crushed

6 kalamata olives, pitted

3 anchovy fillets, finely sliced
    lengthways

Method

1. Cook the potatoes in a saucepan of boiling water for 10–15 minutes or until tender, adding the beans for the last 2 minutes of cooking. Drain and refresh under cold running water. Cut the potatoes in half.

2. Meanwhile, cook the eggs in a small saucepan of boiling water for 9 minutes. Drain and set aside to cool, then peel and cut into quarters.

3. Combine the potatoes, beans, salmon, tomatoes and lettuce in a bowl.

4. Whisk together the vinegar, olive oil, mustard and garlic in a small bowl.

5. Drizzle the dressing over the salad and gently toss to combine. Divide between two bowls.

6. Scatter the olives and anchovies over the salads and top with the egg. Season with freshly ground black pepper and serve.

308 Calories   **12.2 g** Carbs

Nutritional Information
(per serve)

Calories	**308**
Protein	**26.5 g**
Fat Total	**16.2 g**
Fat Saturated	**3.6 g**
Carbohydrates	**12.2 g**
Sugars	**4.8 g**
Sodium	**754.6 mg**
Dietary Fibre	**5.3 g**

Mish Tips

If you are not a fan of anchovies, I urge you to try them from time to time. I used to hate them but they have grown on me. They add so much flavour to a dish, though a little goes a long way!

Less than 20 grams of carbs

Smoky vegetable and haloumi kebabs with lemony rocket salad

Haloumi is a delicious salty cheese that holds its shape when cooked, so it works perfectly in this recipe. Don't cut the pieces too small or they will split in half when you thread them onto the skewers.

Serves: **1** · Prep time: **15 minutes** · Cooking time: **10 minutes** · Great for: *Weekend Lunch*

284 Calories   10.9 g Carbs

Ingredients

1 zucchini, thickly sliced
½ red capsicum, seeded and cut into squares
60 g button mushrooms, halved
½ red onion, cut into wedges
75 g haloumi, cut into 2.5 cm cubes
pinch of smoked paprika
pinch of dried oregano
finely grated zest and juice of ½ lemon
olive oil spray
20 g baby rocket leaves

Method

1. Preheat the grill to medium–high and line a baking tray with foil.

2. Thread the zucchini, capsicum, mushroom, onion and haloumi onto skewers.

3. Combine the paprika, oregano, lemon zest and half the lemon juice in a bowl. Brush over the kebabs, and arrange on the prepared tray. Lightly spray the kebabs with olive oil.

4. Cook under the grill, turning regularly, for 10 minutes or until the vegetables are tender and the haloumi is golden.

5. Toss the rocket and remaining lemon juice in a bowl. Serve with the skewers.

Nutritional Information

(per serve)

Calories	**284**
Protein	**22.1 g**
Fat Total	**14.9 g**
Fat Saturated	**8.4 g**
Carbohydrates	**10.9 g**
Sugars	**10.8 g**
Sodium	**2199.2 mg**
Dietary Fibre	**6.6 g**

Mish Tips

If using wooden or bamboo skewers, soak them in cold water for 15 minutes before threading the food on, to stop them burning during cooking. Vary the vegetables according to what you have on hand. Cherry tomatoes, baby corn and eggplant all work well. Cut the remaining lemon half into wedges and serve on the side, if you like.

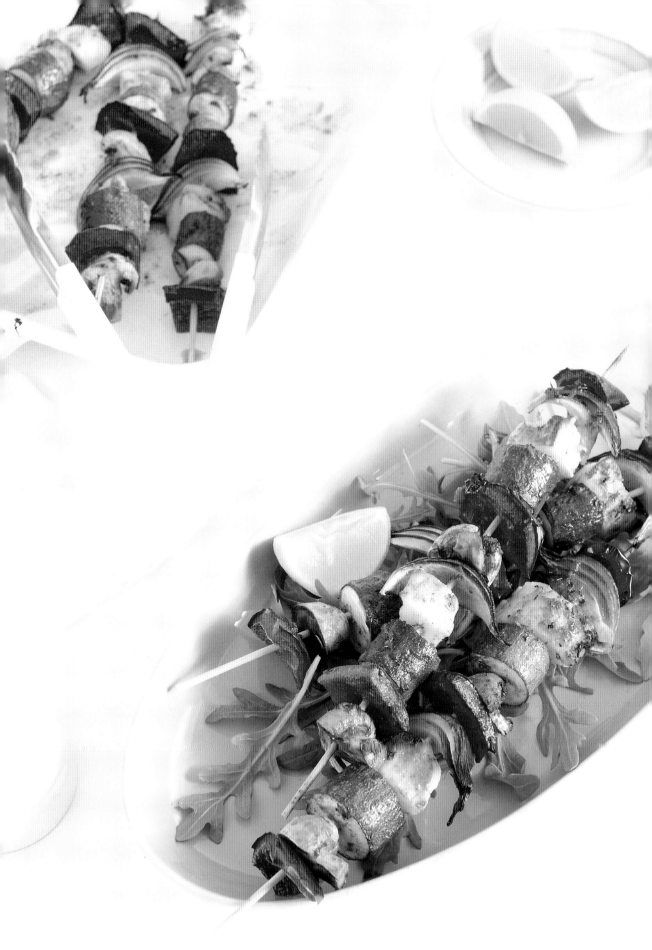

Kangaroo with mint yoghurt and pea salad

Kangaroo is a very lean meat so take care not to overcook it or it will be dry. Resting the meat after cooking helps to retain moisture.

Serves: **2** · Prep time: **20 minutes** · Cooking time: **10 minutes** · Great for: *Dinner*

Ingredients

250 g kangaroo fillet
1 teaspoon ground cumin
1 teaspoon sweet paprika
1 teaspoon olive oil
finely grated zest and juice of 1 lemon
2 tablespoons mint leaves
¾ cup low-fat natural yoghurt
1 clove garlic, crushed
1 cup frozen peas
200 g broccoli, cut into small florets
50 g baby rocket leaves

Method

1. Put the kangaroo in a shallow dish. Combine the cumin, paprika, olive oil, lemon zest and 1 tablespoon lemon juice, then rub over the meat to coat evenly.

2. Finely chop one-quarter of the mint leaves and place in a small bowl. Add the yoghurt and garlic and mix together well. Set aside.

3. Cook the peas and broccoli in a steamer set over a saucepan of simmering water for 3 minutes or until tender but still bright green. Transfer to a bowl and toss with the remaining lemon juice. Allow to cool slightly, then add add the rocket and remaining mint leaves.

4. Meanwhile, heat a non-stick chargrill pan over medium–high heat. Cook the kangaroo for 3 minutes each side for medium. Transfer to a plate and rest for 5 minutes before slicing.

5. Divide the vegetables between two plates and top with the sliced kangaroo. Finish with a dollop of mint yoghurt and serve.

293	13.7 g
Calories	Carbs

Nutritional Information
(per serve)

Calories	**293**
Protein	**41.6 g**
Fat Total	**5.1 g**
Fat Saturated	**0.9 g**
Carbohydrates	**13.7 g**
Sugars	**9.4 g**
Sodium	**171.1 mg**
Dietary Fibre	**11.0 g**

Mish Tips

If you have time, marinate the kangaroo for an hour in the fridge.

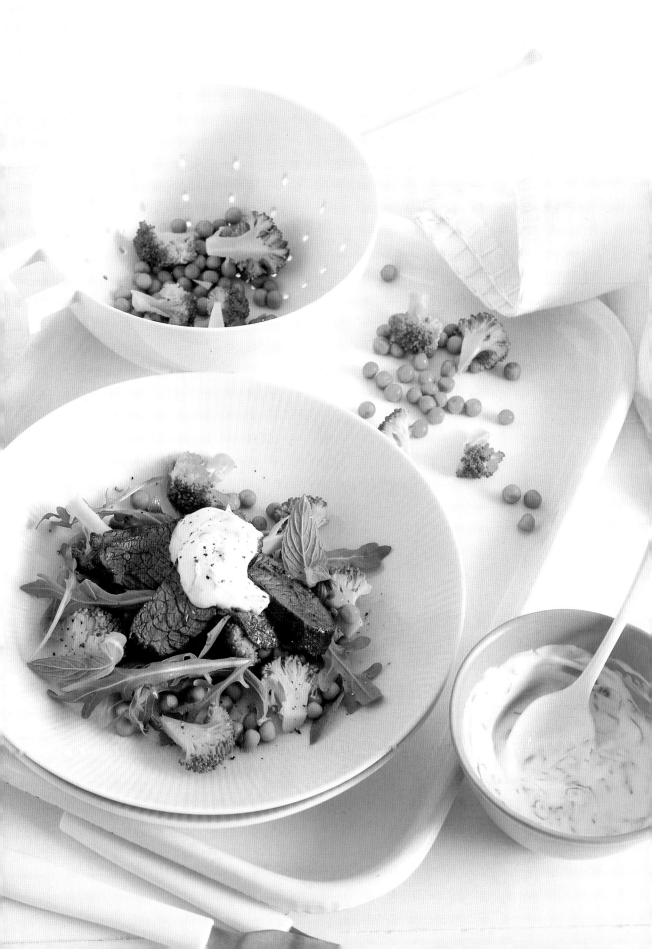

Chicken, lentil and kale soup

You know, you really can make wholesome chicken soup in just 30 minutes. Here's how.

Serves: **2** · Prep time: **15 minutes** · Cooking time: **15 minutes** · Great for: *Lunch, Dinner or Leftovers*

Ingredients

1 teaspoon olive oil

½ leek, white part only, finely sliced

1 carrot, finely sliced

1 celery stalk, finely sliced

250 g lean chicken breast fillet, finely sliced

1 litre salt-reduced chicken stock

150 g kale, stalks removed, leaves shredded

½ cup drained and rinsed tinned lentils

2 tablespoons finely grated parmesan

Method

1. Heat the olive oil in a large saucepan over medium–high heat. Add the leek, carrot, celery and chicken and cook, stirring often, for 4 minutes or until the vegetables start to soften and the chicken changes colour.

2. Pour in the stock and bring to the boil, then reduce the heat to medium–low and simmer, covered, for 5 minutes. Add the kale and simmer for a further 5 minutes.

3. Stir in the lentils and season with freshly ground black pepper. Ladle into bowls, sprinkle with the parmesan and serve.

285	13.9 g
Calories	Carbs

Nutritional Information
(per serve)

Calories	**285**
Protein	**38.9 g**
Fat Total	**7.4 g**
Fat Saturated	**2.8 g**
Carbohydrates	**13.9 g**
Sugars	**10.9 g**
Sodium	**1583.9 mg**
Dietary Fibre	**4.4 g**

Mish Tips

If you don't have any leeks in your pantry, use half a brown onion instead. Replace the lentils with tinned beans or chickpeas if you like – just adjust the calories. To reduce the sodium content you can swap the stock for bone broth.

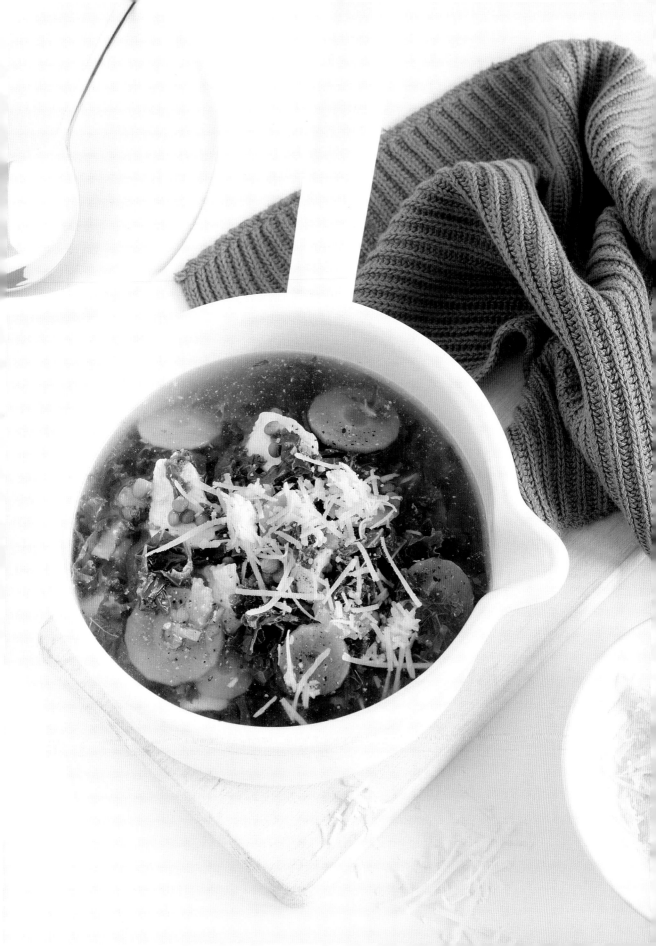

Pork with grape and cabbage salad

This is perfect for a quick dinner. The sweet grapes pair beautifully with the pork, but you could also use cherries or chopped peaches if you like.

Serves: **2** · Prep time: **15 minutes** · Cooking time: **5 minutes** · Great for: *Dinner*

Ingredients

2 x 125 g lean pork butterfly steaks
1 teaspoon wholegrain mustard
olive oil spray
80 g white cabbage, shredded
100 g seedless red grapes, halved
1 celery stalk, sliced
1 carrot, shredded
1 spring onion, sliced
2 teaspoons red wine vinegar
2 teaspoons olive oil
1 tablespoon flaked almonds, toasted

Method

1. Trim any fat from the pork. Rub both sides with the mustard and lightly spray with olive oil. Heat a non-stick frying pan over medium–high heat. Add the pork and cook for 1½ minutes each side or until cooked to your liking. Transfer to a plate, cover loosely with foil and rest for 2 minutes.

2. Meanwhile, combine the cabbage, grapes, celery, carrot and spring onion in a large bowl. Drizzle with the vinegar and olive oil and toss to combine. Season with freshly ground black pepper.

3. Slice the pork and divide between two plates, along with the salad. Sprinkle with the flaked almonds and serve.

287	12.2 g
Calories	Carbs

Nutritional Information
(per serve)

Calories	**287**
Protein	**33.0 g**
Fat Total	**11.0 g**
Fat Saturated	**1.6 g**
Carbohydrates	**12.2 g**
Sugars	**11.8 g**
Sodium	**168.8 mg**
Dietary Fibre	**5.0 g**

You can use pork medallions instead of butterfly steaks if you prefer. They are a little thicker so cook them for 2½ minutes each side.

Tomato *fish stew*

This hearty fish stew is so good even the fussiest of eaters will enjoy it.

Serves: **2** · Prep time: **15 minutes** · Cooking time: **20 minutes** · Great for: *Dinner*

Ingredients

2 teaspoons olive oil

1 leek, white part only, chopped

1 baby fennel bulb, trimmed and finely sliced

1 zucchini, chopped

1 teaspoon vegetable stock powder

1 x 400 g tin diced tomatoes

2 teaspoons dried mixed herbs

350 g white fish fillets, skin and bones removed, cut into 2–3 cm pieces

½ cup drained and rinsed tinned cannellini beans

2 tablespoons chopped flat-leaf parsley

Method

1. Heat the olive oil in a large heavy-based saucepan over medium heat. Add the leek and fennel and cook, stirring, for 3 minutes or until softened. Add the zucchini and cook for 2 minutes.

2. Stir in the stock powder, tomatoes, mixed herbs and 1 cup water. Bring to the boil, then reduce the heat to low and simmer, covered, for 10 minutes.

3. Add the fish and cannellini beans and simmer, covered, for a further 5 minutes or until the fish is cooked and the sauce has thickened slightly. Stir in most of the parsley (save a bit for the top) and season with freshly ground black pepper. Serve sprinkled with the reserved parsley.

318 Calories   17.8 g Carbs

Nutritional Information
(per serve)

Calories	**318**
Protein	**35.2 g**
Fat Total	**9.5 g**
Fat Saturated	**1.8 g**
Carbohydrates	**17.8 g**
Sugars	**12.1 g**
Sodium	**675.5 mg**
Dietary Fibre	**11.5 g**

Mish Tips

If your fennel bulb has any leafy tops, chop them up and sprinkle them on top as a garnish.

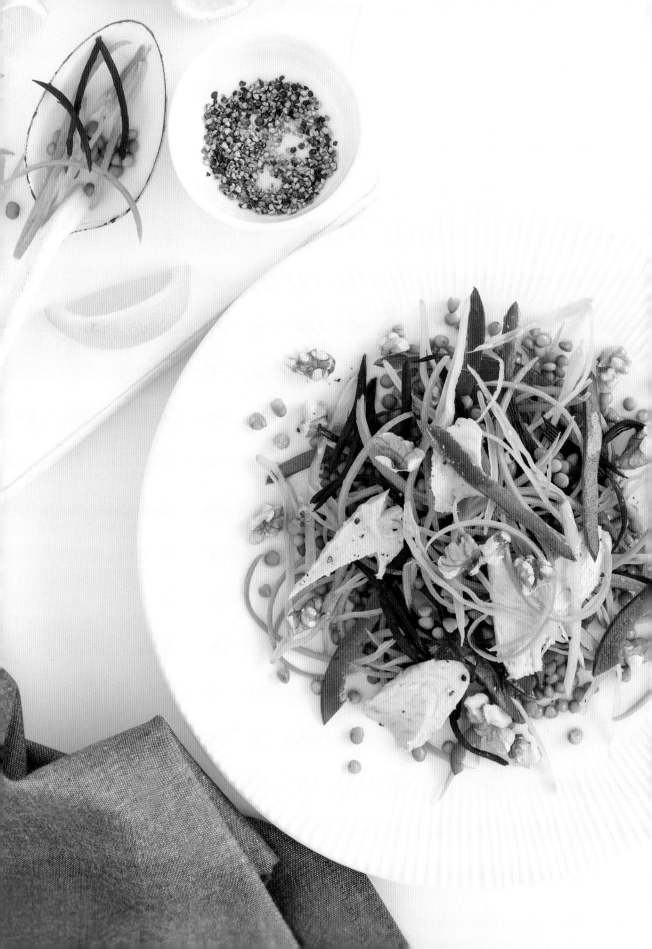

Rainbow *vegetable* salad

When I was growing up, my mum always told us to 'eat rainbows' as that's the best way to get a great range of nutrients into our diets. Mum was right of course, and this recipe always makes me think of her.

Serves: **2** · Prep time: **15 minutes** · Great for: *Lunch*

Ingredients

1 carrot, shredded

100 g snow peas, shredded

100 g beetroot, peeled and shredded

1 red capsicum, seeded and finely sliced

80 g drained and rinsed tinned lentils

40 g walnuts, chopped

2 x 95 g tins tuna in spring water, drained and flaked

1 tablespoon lemon juice

1 teaspoon honey

Method

1. Place the vegetables, lentils, walnuts and tuna in a large bowl.

2. Whisk together the lemon juice and honey in a jug and season well with freshly ground black pepper. Pour over the salad, toss to combine and serve.

323 Calories   **17.1** g Carbs

Nutritional Information
(per serve)

Calories	**323**
Protein	**24.7 g**
Fat Total	**16.0 g**
Fat Saturated	**1.5 g**
Carbohydrates	**17.1 g**
Sugars	**13.5 g**
Sodium	**444.3 mg**
Dietary Fibre	**6.9 g**

Mish Tips

Tinned smoked tuna slices also work well in this recipe. This is a great salad to take to work for lunch. Pack the salad and dressing separately into airtight containers and keep chilled until you're ready to eat.

Roast lamb with lemon, garlic and rosemary

Nothing says Australia like lamb. Paired with rosemary and garlic, this one is sure to be a winner when you're cooking for the masses!

Serves: **10** · Prep time: **20 minutes** · Cooking time: **45 minutes** · Great for: *Weekend Lunch or Dinner*

275	17.7 g
Calories	Carbs

Ingredients

2 cloves garlic, crushed

2 tablespoons chopped rosemary

2 tablespoons olive oil

finely grated zest and juice of 1 lemon

1 x 2 kg boned leg of lamb, tied

1 kg small sweet potatoes, washed, skin left on, halved lengthways

olive oil spray

100 g salad leaves

4 tomatoes, sliced

3 Lebanese cucumbers, sliced

Method

1. Preheat the oven to 200°C (180°C fan-forced). Alternatively, you can use a barbecue with a hood. If you do this, make sure you use a rack so the meat isn't sitting directly on the heat.

2. Combine the garlic, rosemary, olive oil, lemon zest and juice in a small bowl.

3. Place the lamb in a roasting tin. Using a sharp knife, make a few long shallow slits over the top, then spread the rosemary mixture over the lamb. Add the sweet potato to the tin. Lightly spray the lamb and sweet potato with olive oil and season with freshly ground black pepper. Roast for 40–45 minutes or until the meat is cooked to your liking and the sweet potato is tender.

4. Toss together the salad leaves, tomato and cucumber.

5. Slice the lamb and serve with the sweet potato and salad.

Nutritional Information

(per serve)

Calories	**275**
Protein	**27.7 g**
Fat Total	**9.3 g**
Fat Saturated	**3.2 g**
Carbohydrates	**17.7 g**
Sugars	**9.0 g**
Sodium	**112.0 mg**
Dietary Fibre	**5.1 g**

Mish Tips

Using a boned leg of lamb takes the angst out of carving. Ask your butcher to remove the bone and tie the meat for you, or simply purchase one that has been pre-boned in your local supermarket meat department.

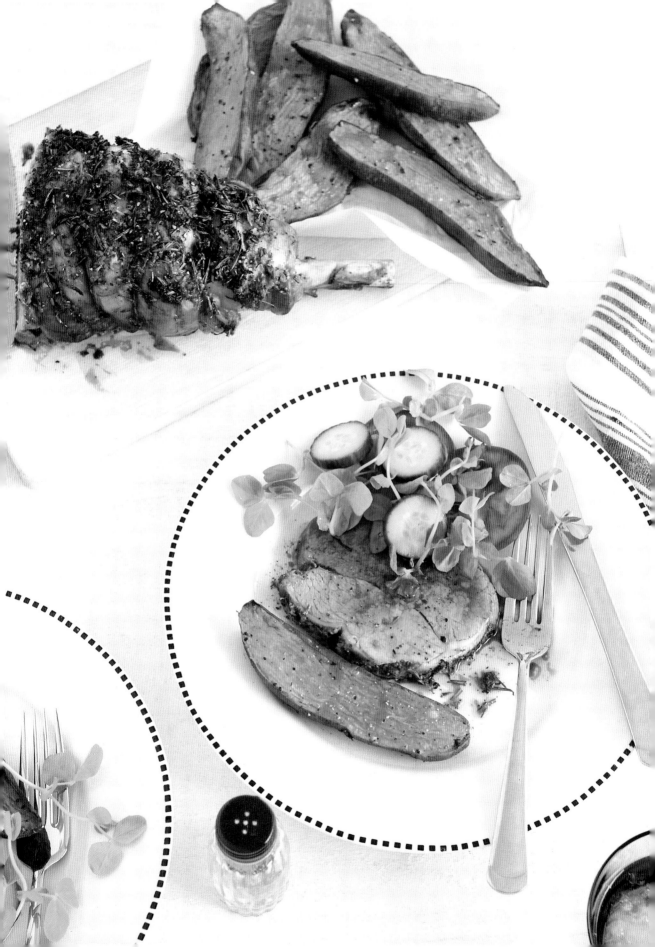

Kale, macadamia and tomato salad with avocado dressing

Kale is a true super food. Combining it with other nutritional powerhouses, macadamias and avocado, means this salad is supercharged!

Serves: **2** • Prep time: **20 minutes** • Great for: *Lunch*

Ingredients

100 g kale, stalks removed, leaves shredded

1 tomato, finely sliced

30 g macadamias, roughly chopped

1 zucchini, cut into ribbons

80 g avocado

100 g low-fat Greek-style yoghurt

1 tablespoon lemon juice

pinch of dried chilli flakes

Method

1. Place the kale, tomato, macadamias and zucchini in a large bowl and toss to combine. Arrange on serving plates. Season with freshly ground black pepper.

2. Place the avocado, yoghurt, lemon juice and chilli flakes in a small food processor (or use a hand-held blender) and blitz until smooth.

3. Drizzle the avocado dressing over the salad and serve.

295	12.3 g
Calories	Carbs

Nutritional Information

(per serve)

Calories	**295**
Protein	**6.7 g**
Fat Total	**23.4 g**
Fat Saturated	**5.5 g**
Carbohydrates	**12.3 g**
Sugars	**12.1 g**
Sodium	**51.2 mg**
Dietary Fibre	**4.9 g**

Mish Tips

Use a vegetable peeler to cut the zucchini into ribbons. If you are unable to find kale, baby spinach or rocket leaves also work well in this salad.

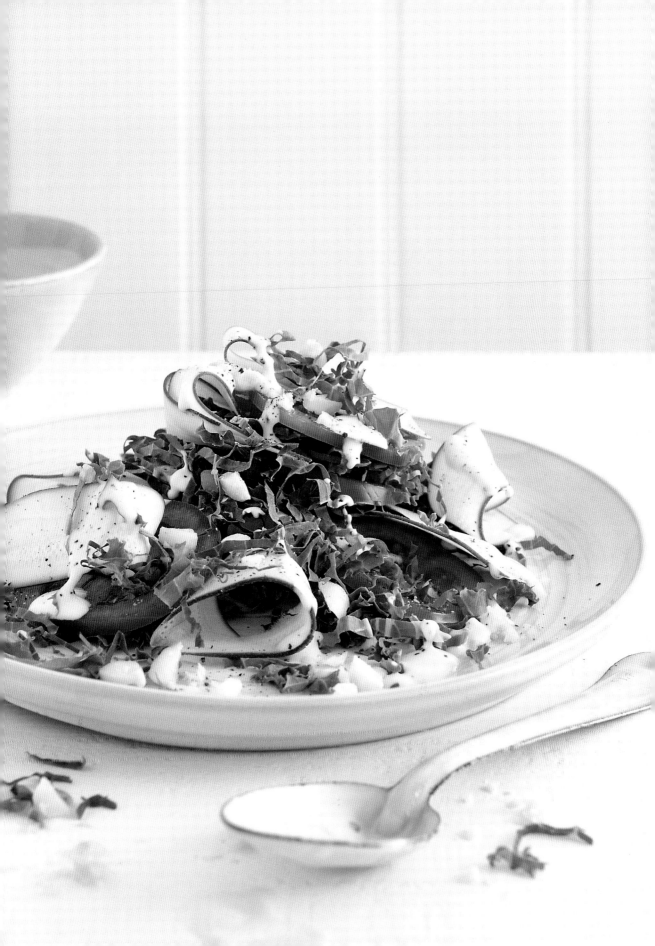

Low-FODMAP *pumpkin* and *spinach lasagne*

Another recipe that proves a low-FODMAP diet doesn't have to be restrictive or boring!

Serves: **2** · Prep time: **20 minutes** · Cooking time: **30 minutes** · Great for: *Lunch, Dinner or Leftovers*

288
Calories

18 g
Carbs

Ingredients

75 g baby spinach leaves
boiling water, for blanching
150 g peeled pumpkin, chopped
100 g drained and rinsed tinned lentils
½ cup basil leaves, chopped
160 g passata
20 kalamata olives, pitted and
    finely sliced
1 eggplant, finely sliced lengthways
1 small zucchini, finely sliced
    lengthways
2 tablespoons finely grated
    low-fat cheddar
1 tablespoon pine nuts

Method

1. Preheat the oven to 180°C (160°C fan-forced).

2. Place the spinach in a heatproof bowl and cover with boiling water to wilt. Drain and refresh under cold running water, then drain well. Squeeze out any excess water and finely chop.

3. Boil, steam or microwave the pumpkin until tender. Drain and mash until smooth, then set aside to cool.

4. Place the spinach, pumpkin, lentils and half the basil in a bowl and mix well. Combine the passata, olives and remaining basil in a separate bowl. Spoon one-third of the passata mixture into the base of two 2-cup capacity baking dishes.

5. Place a thin layer of eggplant and zucchini strips in each dish (these take the place of regular pasta sheets), top with half the pumpkin filling and spread out evenly. Spoon over half the remaining passata mixture. Repeat the layers with the remaining eggplant and zucchini, pumpkin filling and passata mixture. Sprinkle the cheese over the top and bake for 20 minutes or until golden and bubbling. Stand for 5 minutes, then sprinkle with the pine nuts and serve.

Nutritional Information
(per serve)

Calories	**288**
Protein	**10.3 g**
Fat Total	**18.3 g**
Fat Saturated	**2.7 g**
Carbohydrates	**18.0 g**
Sugars	**11.6 g**
Sodium	**951.9 mg**
Dietary Fibre	**7.2 g**

Mish Tips

Use Japanese pumpkin as it has no detectable FODMAPs. Tinned lentils are low FODMAP. Rinse them thoroughly and stick with the specified gram weight.

Spicy chicken and broccoli stir-fry

Stir-fries are a staple meal in our house. They're quick to prepare, you can vary the ingredients according to what you have and, best of all, everyone loves them!

Serves: **2** · Prep time: **10 minutes** · Cooking time: **10 minutes** · Great for: *Dinner*

Ingredients

2 teaspoons olive oil

250 g lean chicken breast fillet, finely sliced

½ red onion, cut into thin wedges

2 cloves garlic, finely sliced

1 teaspoon finely grated ginger

250 g broccoli, cut into florets

1 red capsicum, seeded and finely sliced

100 g sugar snap peas, trimmed

1½ tablespoons hoisin sauce

2 teaspoons sweet chilli sauce

Method

1. Heat 1 teaspoon olive oil in a wok or large non-stick frying pan over high heat. Add the chicken and stir-fry for 2–3 minutes or until golden. Remove to a plate and set aside.

2. Heat the remaining oil in the wok, add the onion and stir-fry for 2 minutes or until golden. Add the garlic and ginger and stir-fry for 30 seconds or until aromatic. Toss in the broccoli, capsicum, sugar snap peas and 1 tablespoon water and stir-fry for 2–3 minutes or until almost tender.

3. Return the chicken to the wok, add the hoisin and sweet chilli sauce and stir-fry for 1 minute or until well coated and heated through. Divide between two plates or bowls and serve.

298 Calories   **13.2 g** Carbs

Nutritional Information
(per serve)

Calories	**298**
Protein	**36.9 g**
Fat Total	**8.7 g**
Fat Saturated	**1.5 g**
Carbohydrates	**13.2 g**
Sugars	**10.9 g**
Sodium	**386.5 mg**
Dietary Fibre	**9.1 g**

Mish Tips

The level of heat in a chilli sauce can really vary between brands, so if you're not sure, start with 1 teaspoon, then add the remainder to taste. Store unpeeled ginger in an airtight bag in the fridge for up to 2 weeks. You could also use grated ginger from a jar if that's more convenient.

Less than 20 grams of carbs

Carrot and asparagus noodles with coriander and coconut dressing

A tropical tasty dish that always makes me think of warm days, swimming and sunbathing on a summer holiday.

Serves: **2** · Prep time: **20 minutes** · Great for: *Weekend Lunch*

Ingredients

1 tablespoon coriander leaves

1 small red chilli, seeded and
    roughly chopped

30 g natural almonds, roughly chopped

3 tablespoons desiccated coconut,
    lightly toasted

2 teaspoons lime juice

1 teaspoon brown sugar

3 tablespoons low-fat coconut milk

2 teaspoons sesame oil

2 carrots, peeled

12 asparagus spears, trimmed

1 tablespoon currants

Method

1. Place the coriander, chilli, half the almonds and 2 tablespoons desiccated coconut in a food processor and blitz until finely chopped. Add the lime juice, sugar, coconut milk and sesame oil. Process again to achieve a pesto-like consistency.

2. Use a vegetable peeler to shave the carrots and asparagus into long thin strips. Place the vegetable 'noodles' in a large bowl.

3. Add the coriander dressing, currants and remaining desiccated coconut to the 'noodles' and gently toss to combine. Sprinkle with the remaining almonds and serve.

303	16 g
Calories	Carbs

Nutritional Information

(per serve)

Calories	**303**
Protein	**7.9 g**
Fat Total	**21.9 g**
Fat Saturated	**8.8 g**
Carbohydrates	**16.0 g**
Sugars	**15.6 g**
Sodium	**41.0 mg**
Dietary Fibre	**9.3 g**

Mish Tips

To toast the coconut, place it in a dry frying pan over medium heat and stir for 1–2 minutes or until lightly golden. Transfer to a plate to cool.

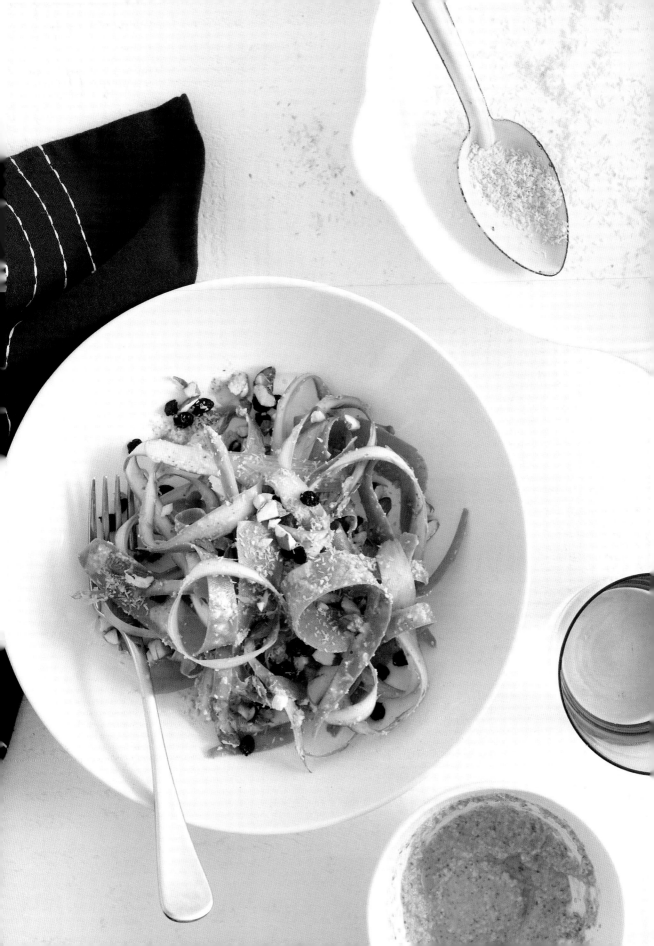

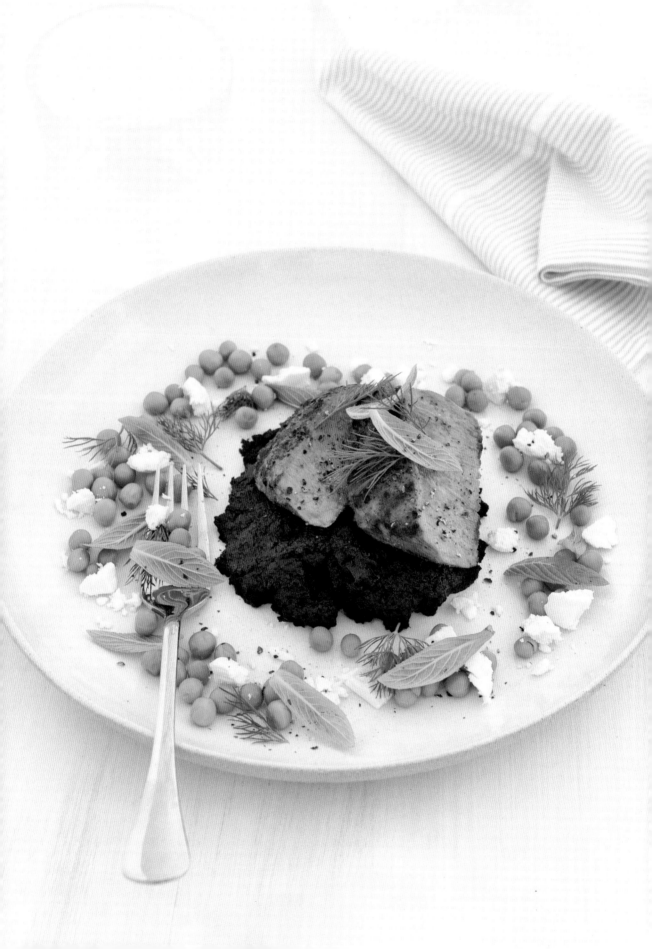

Lamb with beetroot puree and herbed peas

You can't go past fresh beetroot when it's in season, and it works so well with feta and lamb. When it's not in season, use drained tinned baby beetroot.

Serves: **2** • Prep time: **20 minutes** • Cooking time: **55 minutes** • Great for: *Dinner*

Ingredients

1 medium beetroot
olive oil spray
1 teaspoon ground cumin
300 g lamb loin fillet, trimmed
1 cup frozen peas
30 g low-fat feta, crumbled
2 tablespoons mint leaves
1 tablespoon dill leaves

Method

1. Preheat the oven to 220°C (200°C fan-forced). Wrap the beetroot in foil and place on a baking tray. Roast for 45 minutes or until tender, then set aside to cool slightly.

2. Unwrap the beetroot, slip off the skin and roughly chop, then place in a food processor and process to a coarse puree. Season with freshly ground black pepper. Cover and keep warm.

3. Lightly spray a chargrill pan or non-stick frying pan with olive oil and heat over medium–high heat. Sprinkle the cumin on both sides of the lamb and cook for 4 minutes each side for medium, or until cooked to your liking. Transfer to a plate, cover loosely with foil and set aside to rest.

4. Cook the peas in a small saucepan of boiling water until just tender. Drain and return to the pan. Add the feta, mint and dill, season with freshly ground black pepper and toss to combine.

5. Thickly slice the lamb. Divide the beetroot puree between two plates, top with the lamb and scatter around the herbed pea mixture and serve.

294	10.7 g
Calories	Carbs

Nutritional Information

(per serve)

Calories	**294**
Protein	**38.8 g**
Fat Total	**9.3 g**
Fat Saturated	**4.9 g**
Carbohydrates	**10.7 g**
Sugars	**7.6 g**
Sodium	**309.9 mg**
Dietary Fibre	**7.6 g**

Mish Tips

To avoid staining your hands, hold the foil-wrapped beetroot in your hands and use the foil to rub off the skin. Alternatively, use prep gloves.

Less than 20 grams of carbs

Hoisin beef stir-fry with spring vegetables

Yet another of my many stir-fry combinations. Hoisin sauce adds a classic Asian flavour that everyone in the family will enjoy!

Serves: **2** · Prep time: **20 minutes** · Cooking time: **10 minutes** · Great for: *Dinner*

Ingredients

1 teaspoon olive oil

300 g lean rump steak, finely sliced

½ bunch asparagus, trimmed and sliced

2 yellow squash, finely sliced

½ bunch broccolini, cut into separate stems and tops

100 g snow peas, halved diagonally

1 clove garlic, finely chopped

1½ tablespoons salt-reduced soy sauce

1½ tablespoons hoisin sauce

Method

1. Heat half the olive oil in a wok or large non-stick frying pan over high heat. Working in batches, stir-fry the beef for 1 minute or until browned. Transfer to a plate.

2. Heat the remaining oil in the wok. Add the asparagus, squash and broccolini stems and stir-fry for 2 minutes. Add the snow peas, broccolini tops and 2 teaspoons water and stir-fry for 2 minutes or until all the vegetables are tender but still crisp.

3. Return the beef to the wok, along with the garlic and sauces, and stir-fry for 1 minute or until heated through. Serve immediately.

312	12.4 g
Calories	Carbs

Nutritional Information
(per serve)

Calories	**312**
Protein	**38.9 g**
Fat Total	**10.7 g**
Fat Saturated	**3.1 g**
Carbohydrates	**12.4 g**
Sugars	**10.4 g**
Sodium	**817.8 mg**
Dietary Fibre	**6.6 g**

Mish Tips

If you would like to make this vegetarian, simply replace the beef with firm tofu.

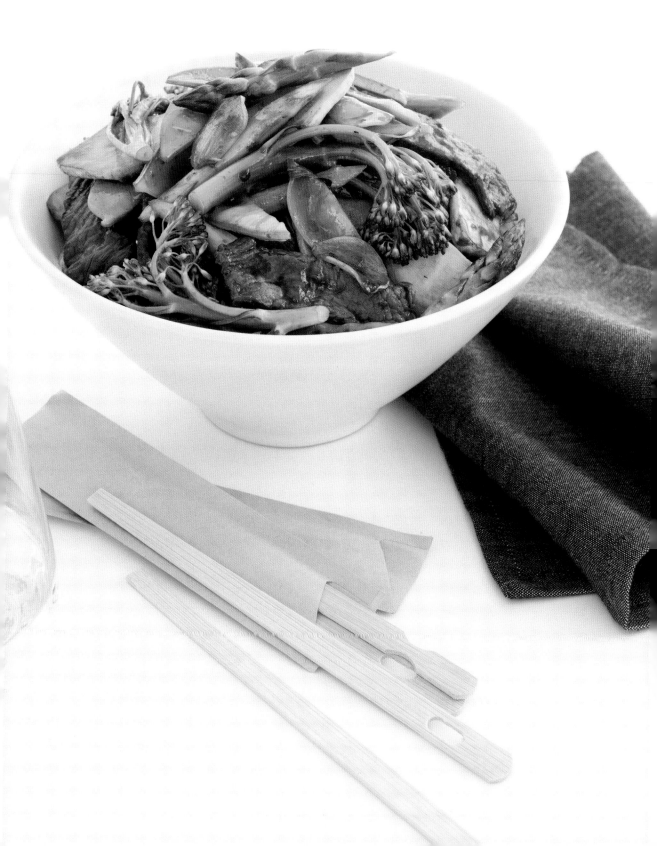

Potato, spinach and feta tortilla

This tasty tortilla is packed with veggies and protein – great for brunch, lunch or an easy evening meal.

Serves: **2** • Prep time: **10 minutes** • Cooking time: **30 minutes** • Great for: *Breakfast, Lunch or Dinner*

Ingredients

180 g potato, roughly chopped

2 teaspoons olive oil

1 red onion, cut into thin wedges

1 red capsicum, seeded and
    roughly chopped

40 g baby spinach leaves

3 cage-free eggs

⅓ cup low-fat milk

40 g low-fat feta, roughly chopped

20 g baby rocket leaves

Method

1. Place the potato in a shallow microwave-safe bowl and add 3 tablespoons water. Cover and microwave on high for 4 minutes or until just tender. Drain well, and set aside to cool slightly.

2. Heat the olive oil in a small ovenproof frying pan over medium–high heat. Add the onion, capsicum and potato and cook, stirring occasionally, for 4 minutes or until the onion is lightly golden and starting to soften. Add the spinach and cook, stirring, for a further minute or until it starts to wilt.

3. Meanwhile, whisk the eggs, milk and some freshly ground black pepper in a small bowl.

4. Pour the egg mixture over the vegetables in the pan, then sprinkle with the feta. Reduce the heat to low and cook for 10 minutes or until the mixture starts to set around the edges.

5. Preheat the grill to medium. Place the pan under the grill and cook for a further 8 minutes or until the egg is golden and set. Remove the pan from the grill and rest for 5 minutes. Cut the tortilla into four pieces. Place two pieces on each plate and serve with the rocket leaves.

327	19 g
Calories	Carbs

Nutritional Information
(per serve)

Calories	**327**
Protein	**22.2 g**
Fat Total	**17.5 g**
Fat Saturated	**7.2 g**
Carbohydrates	**19.0 g**
Sugars	**7.2 g**
Sodium	**382.7 mg**
Dietary Fibre	**3.7 g**

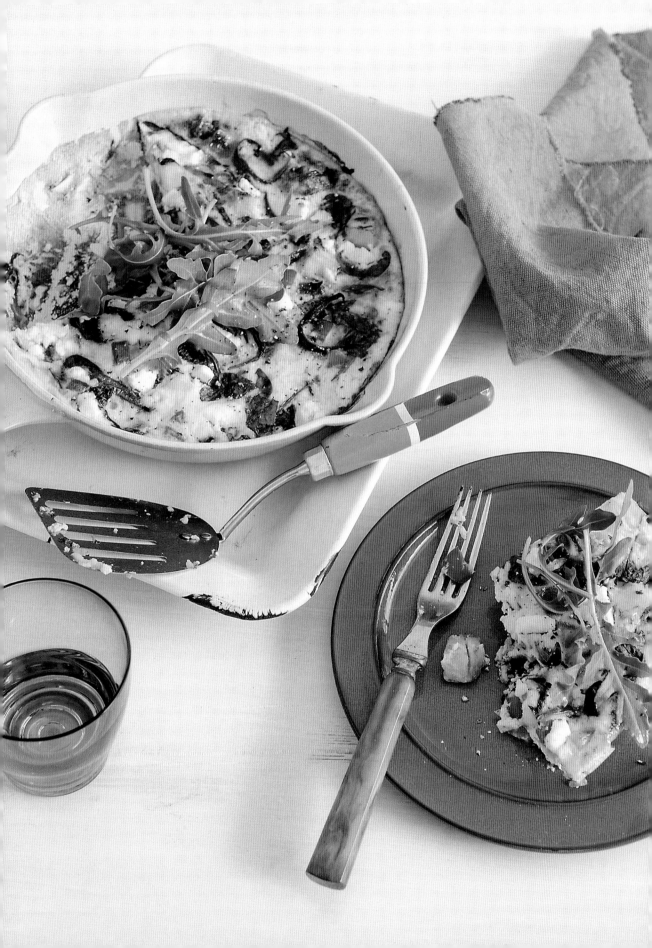

Chicken and vegetables in coconut

This creamy, fragrant dish has a divine flavour without the heat of a curry. Everyone will love the taste, and the washer-upper will love only having one pan to clean!

Serves: **4** · Prep time: **15 minutes** · Cooking time: **25 minutes** · Great for: *Lunch, Dinner or Leftvers*

311 Calories   **10.7** g Carbs

Ingredients

8 lean chicken drumsticks
olive oil spray
2 teaspoons grated ginger
1 lemongrass stalk, white part only,
    finely chopped
2 cloves garlic, crushed
1 x 160 ml tin low-fat coconut milk
¾ cup salt-reduced chicken stock
2 carrots, chopped
150 g cauliflower, cut into small florets
150 g broccoli, cut into small florets
100 g frozen peas
160 g drained and rinsed
    tinned chickpeas

Method

1. Season the chicken drumsticks with freshly ground black pepper. Lightly spray a large non-stick frying pan with olive oil and heat over medium–high heat. Add the chicken and cook, turning regularly for 5 minutes or until nicely browned.

2. Add the ginger, lemongrass and garlic and cook, stirring, for 30 seconds. Pour in the coconut milk and stock. Reduce the heat to medium and simmer, covered, for 10 minutes.

3. Add the vegetables and chickpeas and simmer for a further 5 minutes or until the veggies are tender and the chicken is cooked through.

4. Divide the chicken, vegetables and chickpeas among bowls. Spoon over the sauce and serve.

Nutritional Information
(per serve)

Calories	**311**
Protein	**36.7 g**
Fat Total	**12.1 g**
Fat Saturated	**5.0 g**
Carbohydrates	**10.7 g**
Sugars	**3.7 g**
Sodium	**432.7 mg**
Dietary Fibre	**7.4 g**

Mish Tips

Low-fat coconut milk turns what could be a crazy high-calorie meal into a controlled and tasty one. Enjoy treating yourself!

Low-FODMAP *steak* with grilled summer veggies

FODMAPs are carbohydrates that tend to 'ferment' in the gut, leading to bloating and tummy discomfort. Here, we've removed onion and garlic from the original recipe for sensitive bellies, but feel free to add some to the barbecue if you love them.

Serves: **2** · Prep time: **10 minutes** · Cooking time: **10 minutes** · Great for: *Dinner*

Ingredients

- 140 g sweet potato, scrubbed and cut into wedges
- 2 teaspoons olive oil
- 1 zucchini, sliced
- 1 red capsicum, seeded and cut into 2 cm thick strips
- 100 g cherry tomatoes
- 250 g beef eye fillet
- olive oil spray
- 20 g baby rocket leaves
- 1 tablespoon balsamic vinegar

Method

1. Place the sweet potato on a plate and cover loosely with plastic film. Microwave on high for 3 minutes or until tender. Drain and set aside to cool slightly.

2. Preheat a barbecue grill to medium–high or heat a chargrill pan over medium–high heat. Lightly drizzle the olive oil over the sweet potato, zucchini, capsicum and tomatoes and cook on the grill, turning once, for 5 minutes or until tender and lightly charred.

3. Meanwhile, lightly spray both sides of the steak with olive oil and add to the grill. Cook for 2 minutes each side for medium, or until cooked to your liking. Transfer to a plate, cover loosely with foil and rest for 2 minutes before slicing.

4. Divide the beef and vegetables between two plates. Add the rocket and drizzle with the balsamic vinegar. Season with freshly ground black pepper and serve.

310	14.7 g
Calories	Carbs

Nutritional Information

(per serve)

Calories	**310**
Protein	**31.2 g**
Fat Total	**13.0 g**
Fat Saturated	**3.4 g**
Carbohydrates	**14.7 g**
Sugars	**8.7 g**
Sodium	**88.5 mg**
Dietary Fibre	**5.0 g**

 Mish Tips

Garlic-infused olive oil can be used for a broader flavour profile. In order to keep this meal low FODMAP, do not exceed 70 g sweet potato per serve.

Less than 20 grams of carbs

Lamb with Moroccan carrot salad

I love tantalising my tastebuds with flavours from all around the globe. The tang of Moroccan flavours combined with good old Aussie lamb is the perfect balance of home and abroad!

Serves: **2** · Prep time: **10 minutes** · Cooking time: **5 minutes** · Great for: *Weekend Lunch or Dinner*

313	19.3 g
Calories	Carbs

Ingredients

1 tablespoon currants

2 tablespoons lemon juice

2 tablespoons low-fat natural yoghurt

2 teaspoons tahini

200 g lean lamb steak

1 teaspoon sumac

olive oil spray

1 carrot, coarsely grated

1 cup drained and rinsed tinned chickpeas

3 tablespoons roughly chopped flat-leaf parsley

Method

1. Combine the currants and 1½ tablespoons lemon juice in a bowl and set aside to soften. Mix the remaining lemon juice with the yoghurt and tahini in a small bowl.

2. Heat a frying pan over medium–high heat. Sprinkle the lamb with ¾ teaspoon sumac and lightly spray with olive oil. Add to the pan and cook for about 2 minutes each side for medium–rare, or until cooked to your liking. Transfer to a plate, cover loosely with foil and rest for a few minutes before slicing.

3. Add the carrot, chickpeas and parsley to the currant mixture and toss to combine.

4. Divide the salad between two plates and top with the sliced lamb and tahini yoghurt. Sprinkle with the remaining sumac and serve.

Nutritional Information

(per serve)

Calories	**313**
Protein	**30.2 g**
Fat Total	**11.4 g**
Fat Saturated	**2.7 g**
Carbohydrates	**19.3 g**
Sugars	**8.1 g**
Sodium	**319.8 mg**
Dietary Fibre	**6.6 g**

Mish Tips

Sumac is a ground dried berry with a vibrant red colour and citrus flavour. It is available in the spice section at the supermarket.

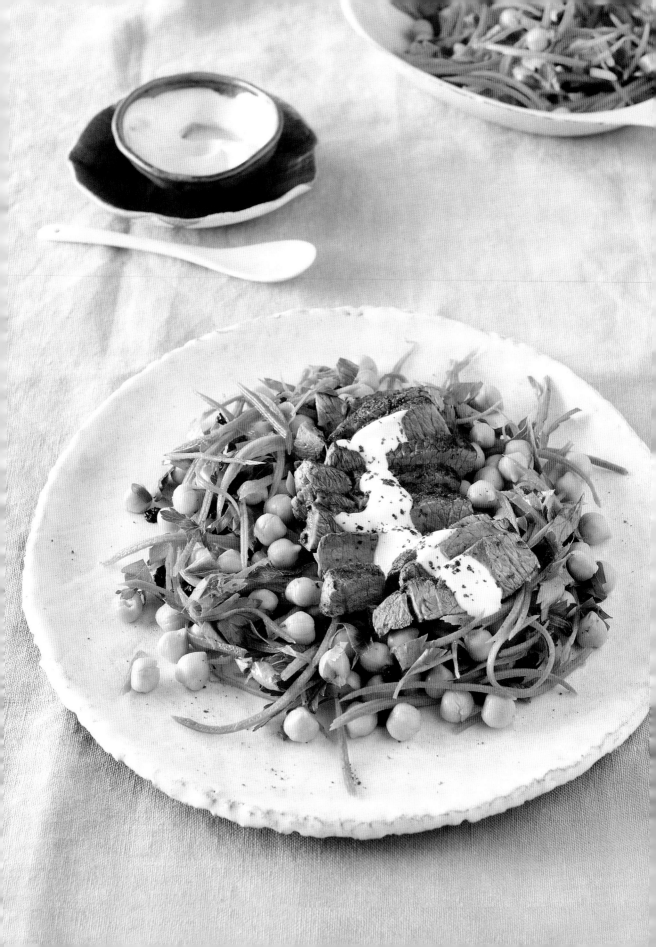

Zucchini cakes with dill raita

Another firm favourite for all the vegetarians out there – golden zucchini cakes with a moreish dill raita.

Serves: **2** • Prep time: **20 minutes** • Cooking time: **10 minutes** • Great for: *Breakfast or Lunch*

Ingredients

2 zucchini, grated
20 g low-fat feta, crumbled
1 spring onion, sliced
⅓ cup quinoa flakes
10 g flaked almonds
1 cage-free egg, lightly beaten
1 teaspoon olive oil
60 g low-fat natural yoghurt
2 teaspoons chopped dill
1 clove garlic, crushed
2 teaspoons tahini
125 g cherry tomatoes, halved
30 g baby rocket leaves

Method

1. Take handfuls of the grated zucchini and squeeze out as much moisture as possible. Combine the zucchini, feta, spring onion, quinoa flakes, flaked almonds and egg in a large bowl and season with freshly ground black pepper.

2. Heat the olive oil in a non-stick frying pan over medium heat. For each zucchini cake, drop 3 tablespoons of the mixture into the pan and flatten slightly with the back of a spoon (depending on the size of your pan you may need to do this in two batches). Cook for 2–3 minutes each side or until lightly golden and cooked through. Remove and cover to keep warm while you cook the remaining cakes (you should have six altogether).

3. Meanwhile, combine the yoghurt, dill, garlic and tahini in a small bowl.

4. Place three zucchini cakes on each plate. Serve with the tomatoes, rocket and dill raita.

266
Calories

16.6 g
Carbs

Nutritional Information

(per serve)

Calories	**266**
Protein	**14.3 g**
Fat Total	**15.0 g**
Fat Saturated	**3.9 g**
Carbohydrates	**16.6 g**
Sugars	**6.7 g**
Sodium	**191.6 mg**
Dietary Fibre	**3.8 g**

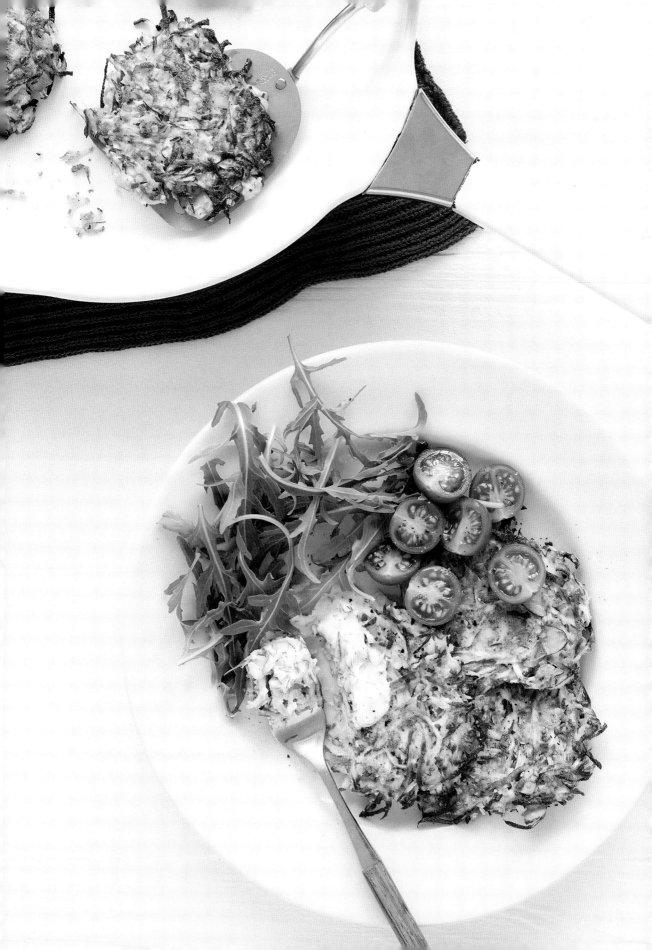

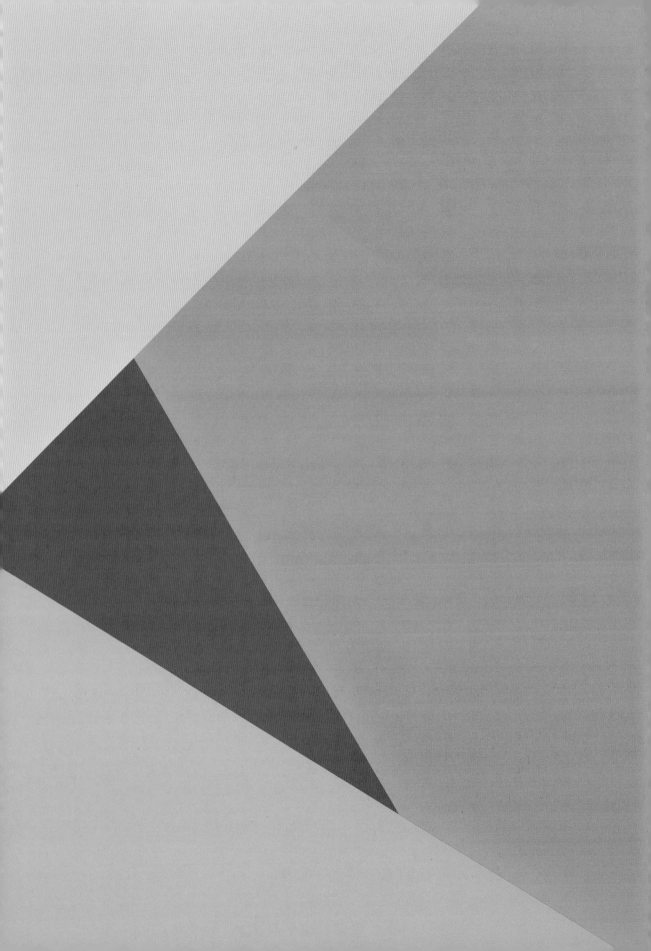

< LESS THAN

30

grams of carbs

Saganaki-style *prawns*

These prawns cooked in a Greek style are quick, easy and delicious!

Serves: **2** · Prep time: **5 minutes** · Cooking time: **15 minutes** · Great for: *Dinner*

Ingredients

olive oil spray

1 red onion, chopped

2 cloves garlic, crushed

1 tablespoon tomato paste

1 x 400 g tin diced tomatoes

1 tablespoon white wine vinegar

250 g raw king prawns, peeled and
    deveined, tails intact

300 g frozen mixed vegetables

20 g low-fat feta

2 tablespoons chopped
    flat-leaf parsley

Method

1. Lightly spray an ovenproof non-stick frying pan with olive oil and heat over medium–high heat. Add the onion and cook, stirring, for 2 minutes. Add the garlic and cook for 30 seconds, then stir in the tomato paste, tomatoes and vinegar and simmer for 3 minutes.

2. Add the prawns and simmer for 3 minutes or until the prawns are just cooked. Add the mixed vegetables and heat through. Season with freshly ground black pepper.

3. Preheat the grill to medium–high and crumble the feta over the prawns. Grill for 2 minutes or until golden. Sprinkle the parsley over the top and serve immediately.

283 Calories   20.6 g Carbs

Nutritional Information

(per serve)

Calories	**283**
Protein	**34.4 g**
Fat Total	**3.6 g**
Fat Saturated	**2.3 g**
Carbohydrates	**20.6 g**
Sugars	**14.9 g**
Sodium	**814.7 mg**
Dietary Fibre	**14.8 g**

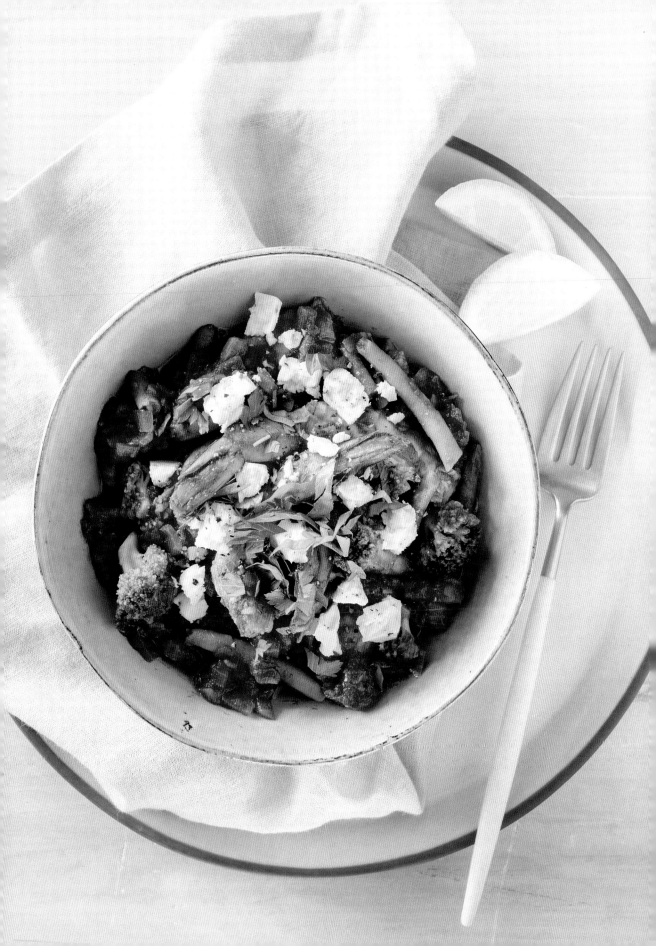

Portuguese *piri piri* chicken with quinoa salad

Piri piri chicken is a hit in our household. We keep a lid on the zing for Axel by preparing his chicken when we make the salad, but for the adults we up the ante by marinating the chicken overnight!

Serves: **2** · Prep time: **15 minutes** · Cooking time: **15 minutes** · Great for: *Dinner*

298	23.2 g
Calories	Carbs

Ingredients

1 small red chilli, seeded and roughly chopped

100 g chargrilled capsicum, ½ roughly chopped, ½ finely sliced

2 cloves garlic, roughly chopped

1 teaspoon sweet or smoked paprika

½ teaspoon dried oregano

2 tablespoons lemon juice

250 g lean chicken breast fillet, cut into thin strips

3 tablespoons red quinoa, rinsed and drained

100 g baby spinach leaves

1 Lebanese cucumber, halved lengthways and finely sliced

Method

1. Place the chilli, chopped capsicum, garlic, paprika, oregano and lemon juice in a food processor and process until smooth. Place the chicken in a glass or ceramic dish. Pour the chilli mixture over the chicken and turn to coat. Cover and marinate in the fridge until required.

2. Cook the quinoa in a saucepan of boiling water for 12 minutes. Drain well and fluff up the grains with a fork.

3. Meanwhile, preheat the grill to high and line a baking tray with foil. Arrange the chicken on the tray and grill, turning once, for 5 minutes or until the chicken is cooked through.

4. Toss the spinach, cucumber, quinoa and sliced capsicum in a bowl. Divide between two plates, top with the chicken and serve.

Nutritional Information
(per serve)

Calories	**298**
Protein	**34.1 g**
Fat Total	**7.5 g**
Fat Saturated	**1.2 g**
Carbohydrates	**23.2 g**
Sugars	**3.8 g**
Sodium	**304.8 mg**
Dietary Fibre	**5.0 g**

Mish Tips

To chargrill a capsicum, cut it into large pieces and remove the seeds and membrane. Place, skin side up, under a hot grill or, skin side down, on a hot chargrill pan and cook until the skin has blistered and blackened. Let it cool, then remove the skin and cut the flesh as required. We used red quinoa here, but you can use white or black if that's what you have. Red and black quinoa generally take a minute or so longer to cook than white.

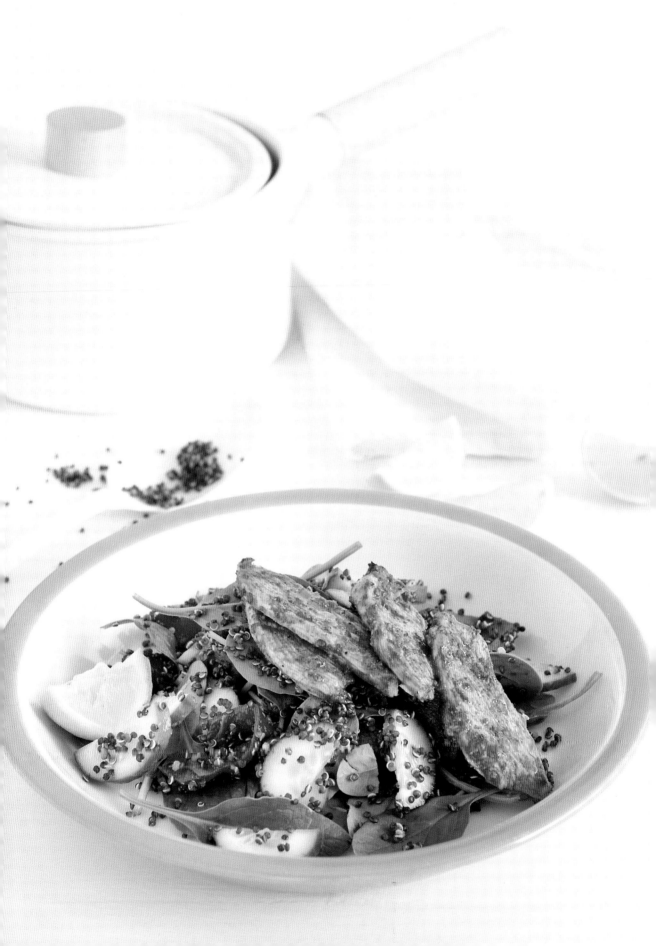

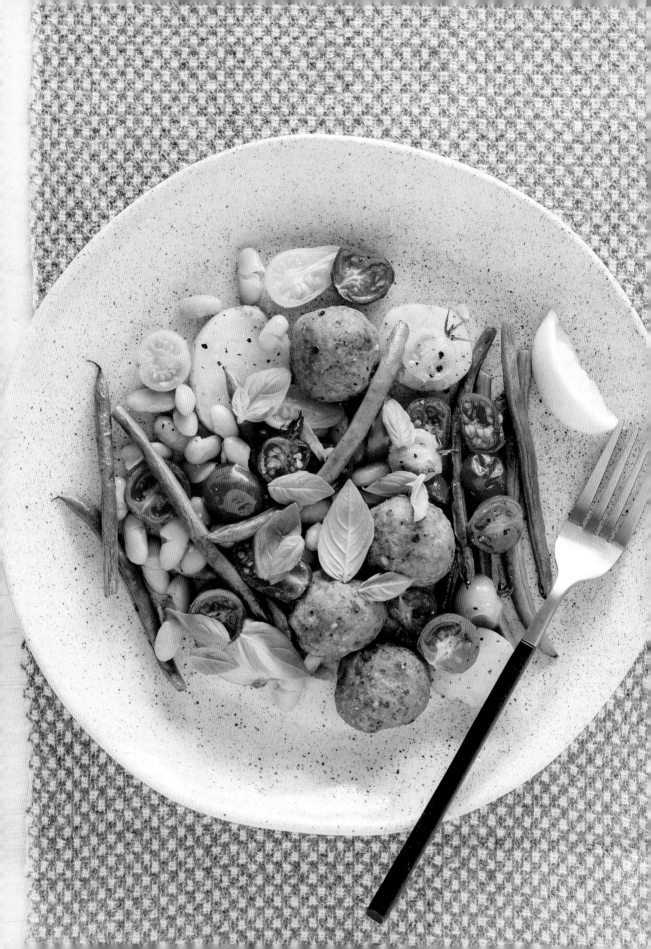

Italian turkey *meatball* tray bake

Just put everything together on a baking tray and pop it in the oven — what could be easier?

Serves: **4** · Prep time: **20 minutes** · Cooking time: **35 minutes** · Great for: *Lunch, Dinner or Leftovers*

Ingredients

500 g turkey mince

3 teaspoons dried oregano

finely grated zest and juice of 1 lemon

300 g potatoes, peeled and cut into
    1 cm thick slices

olive oil spray

250 g green beans, trimmed

1 x 400 g tin cannellini beans, drained
    and rinsed

200 g cherry tomatoes, halved

3 tablespoons baby basil leaves

Method

1. Preheat the oven to 200°C (180°C fan-forced). Line a large baking tray with baking paper.

2. Combine the turkey mince, oregano and lemon zest in a bowl and season with freshly ground black pepper. Roll the mixture into walnut-sized balls.

3. Arrange the potato slices over the prepared tray and add the meatballs. Lightly spray with olive oil and bake for 15 minutes.

4. Add the green beans, cannellini beans and tomatoes to the tray. Increase the temperature to 210°C (190°C fan-forced) and bake for a further 15–20 minutes or until lightly golden and the meatballs are cooked through.

5. Divide the meatballs and vegetables among plates and drizzle with the lemon juice. Scatter over the basil leaves and serve.

286	20.2 g
Calories	Carbs

Nutritional Information

(per serve)

Calories	**286**
Protein	**34.3 g**
Fat Total	**5.1 g**
Fat Saturated	**1.3 g**
Carbohydrates	**20.2 g**
Sugars	**4.1 g**
Sodium	**468.8 mg**
Dietary Fibre	**8.6 g**

Mish Tips

You can replace the dried oregano with mixed dried Italian herbs if preferred. Chicken mince also works well in this recipe.

Braised pumpkin and lentils with haloumi

Mmmm . . . haloumi. It's so good with this hearty pumpkin and lentil braise. Who said vego food was boring?

Serves: **4** · Prep time: **15 minutes** · Cooking time: **25 minutes** · Great for: *Dinner*

302 **Calories**   24.2 g **Carbs**

Ingredients

1 tablespoon olive oil

1 brown onion, finely chopped

2 cloves garlic, crushed

200 g mushrooms, quartered

400 g peeled pumpkin, cut into
1.5 cm cubes

2 x 400 g tins lentils, drained and rinsed

2 x 400 g tins cherry tomatoes

½ cup salt-reduced vegetable stock

2 tablespoons balsamic vinegar

125 g haloumi

40 g baby rocket leaves

Method

1. Heat the olive oil in a large deep non-stick frying pan over medium heat. Add the onion and cook for 5 minutes or until softened. Add the garlic and cook, stirring, for about 30 seconds.

2. Add the mushroom, pumpkin, lentils, tomatoes and stock. Cover and bring to a simmer, then reduce the heat to low and cook gently for 10 minutes. Remove the lid and cook for a further 5 minutes or until the liquid has reduced and the vegetables are tender. Stir in the balsamic vinegar and season with freshly ground black pepper.

3. Cook the haloumi in a non-stick frying pan over medium heat for 1 minute each side or until golden brown.

4. Serve the lentil mixture topped with the warm haloumi and rocket leaves.

Nutritional Information
(per serve)

Calories	**302**
Protein	**18.1 g**
Fat Total	**11.5 g**
Fat Saturated	**4.2 g**
Carbohydrates	**24.2 g**
Sugars	**15.2 g**
Sodium	**1507.9 mg**
Dietary Fibre	**7.0 g**

Mish Tips

If you don't have tinned cherry tomatoes, just use regular diced tomatoes.

Tuna *frittata*

The whole family will love this dish — and if not, it makes perfect leftovers for lunch the next day!

Serves: **4** • Prep time: **15 minutes** • Cooking time: **1 hour** • Great for: *Lunch, Dinner or Leftovers*

Ingredients

½ cup brown rice

olive oil spray

1 red capsicum, seeded and chopped

4 spring onions, sliced

1 x 185 g tin tuna in spring water, drained and flaked

1 zucchini, chopped

100 g frozen corn kernels

⅓ cup low-fat cottage cheese

4 cage-free eggs, lightly beaten

50 g baby spinach leaves

250 g cherry tomatoes, halved

1 lemon, cut into wedges

Method

1. Cook the rice in a saucepan of boiling water for 30 minutes or until tender. Drain well.

2. Meanwhile, preheat the oven to 190°C (170°C fan-forced). Lightly spray a 20 cm square cake tin with olive oil and line with baking paper, extending up two sides to help you lift the frittata out later.

3. Lightly spray a non-stick frying pan with olive oil and heat over medium heat. Add the capsicum and spring onion and cook, stirring occasionally, for 3–4 minutes or until softened. Transfer to a large bowl. Add the tuna, zucchini, corn, cottage cheese, eggs and cooked rice and mix well.

4. Transfer the mixture to the prepared tin and bake for 30 minutes or until set and lightly golden. Cool slightly, then lift the frittata from the tin and cut into four squares. Serve with the spinach leaves and tomatoes, with the lemon wedges on the side.

296 Calories   **28.1 g** Carbs

Nutritional Information

(per serve)

Calories	**296**
Protein	**22.7 g**
Fat Total	**9.7 g**
Fat Saturated	**2.7 g**
Carbohydrates	**28.1 g**
Sugars	**5.3 g**
Sodium	**299.7 mg**
Dietary Fibre	**4.5 g**

Sweet potato and tuna poke bowl

Poke bowls have become hugely popular and for good reason. Enjoy this simple tuna version.

Serves: **2** · Prep time: **10 minutes** · Cooking time: **5 minutes** · Great for: *Lunch*

Ingredients

200 g sweet potato, peeled and cut into 2 cm pieces

100 g cherry tomatoes, quartered

60 g avocado, diced

60 g baby spinach leaves

150 g drained and rinsed tinned four bean mix

2 x 95 g tins tuna in spring water, drained and flaked

3 tablespoons chopped coriander

2 teaspoons balsamic vinegar

Method

1. Place the sweet potato in a microwave-safe bowl and add 3 tablespoons water. Cover and microwave on high for 3 minutes or until tender. Drain and set aside to cool.

2. Arrange the sweet potato, tomato, avocado, spinach, beans and tuna in two serving bowls. Scatter over the coriander and drizzle with the balsamic vinegar. Season with freshly ground black pepper and serve.

301	27 g
Calories	Carbs

Nutritional Information
(per serve)

Calories	**301**
Protein	**24.7 g**
Fat Total	**8.7 g**
Fat Saturated	**2.1 g**
Carbohydrates	**27.0 g**
Sugars	**9.0 g**
Sodium	**564.6 mg**
Dietary Fibre	**10.2 g**

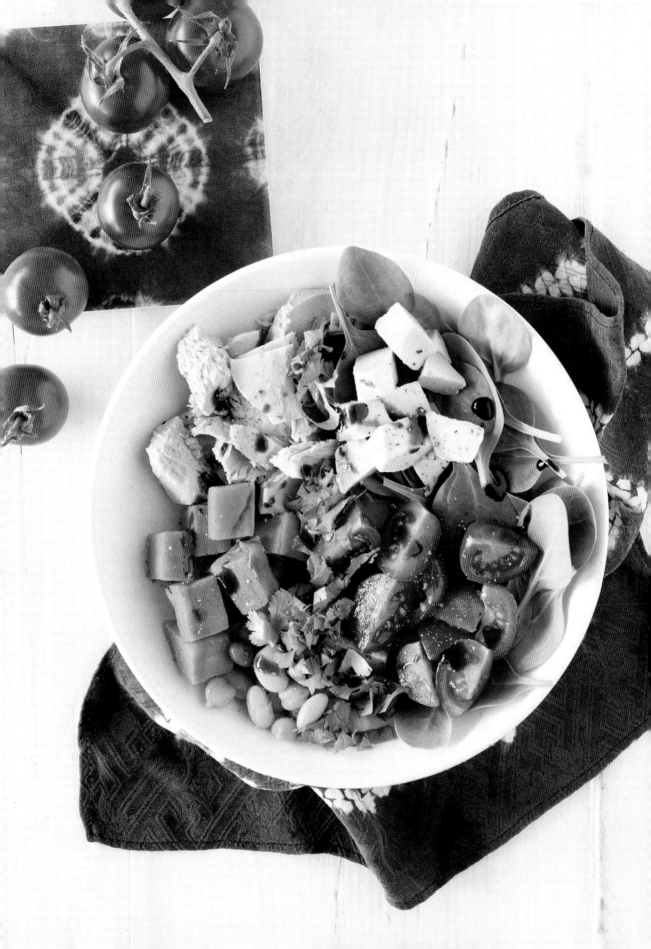

Rainbow salad jar

This is a great take-to-work lunch that you can put together the night before.

Serves: **2** · Prep time: **15 minutes** · Great for: *Lunch*

Ingredients

3 teaspoons olive oil

1½ tablespoons lemon juice

1 cup drained and rinsed tinned black beans

½ beetroot, coarsely grated

1 tomato, chopped

1 carrot, coarsely grated

1 x 125 g tin corn kernels, drained

1 spring onion, sliced

30 g baby spinach leaves

1 tablespoon unsalted pistachio kernels, chopped

Method

1. Divide the olive oil and lemon juice evenly between two 2-cup capacity jars or airtight containers. Season with freshly ground black pepper.

2. Layer the black beans, beetroot, tomato, carrot, corn, spring onion and spinach into the jars and top with the pistachios. Seal tightly and keep refrigerated until serving time.

3. To serve, invert the salads into bowls and toss to mix the dressing through.

301 Calories	**29** g Carbs

Nutritional Information
(per serve)

Calories	**301**
Protein	**13.0 g**
Fat Total	**12.2 g**
Fat Saturated	**1.6 g**
Carbohydrates	**29.0 g**
Sugars	**22.8 g**
Sodium	**163.9 mg**
Dietary Fibre	**13.6 g**

Don't mix up the order of layering!
Keep the dressing at the bottom
and the leaves and nuts at the top to
prevent a soggy salad come lunchtime.

Eggplant, sweet potato and ricotta bake

Everyone loves a good veggie bake and this one is sure to please.

Serves: **4** • Prep time: **30 minutes** • Cooking time: **1 hour 15 minutes** • Great for: *Lunch, Dinner or Leftovers*

292 Calories 27 g Carbs

Ingredients

500 g sweet potato, peeled and cut lengthways into 1 cm thick slices
olive oil spray
500 g eggplant, finely sliced
1 brown onion, chopped
100 g mushrooms, chopped
2 cloves garlic, crushed
300 g fresh low-fat ricotta
75 g basil leaves, chopped
1 x 400 g tin diced tomatoes
50 g low-fat mozzarella, grated
40 g baby spinach leaves

Method

1. Preheat the oven to 200°C (180°C fan-forced). Line a baking tray with baking paper.

2. Place the sweet potato on the prepared tray, lightly spray with olive oil and season with freshly ground black pepper. Bake for 30 minutes or until tender.

3. Meanwhile, lightly spray a large non-stick frying pan with olive oil and heat over medium heat. Add the eggplant in batches and cook for 2–3 minutes each side or until golden. Spray the pan with extra oil as needed. Transfer to a plate and cover to keep warm.

4. Spray a little more oil in the pan. Add the onion, mushroom and garlic and cook, stirring often, for 5 minutes or until soft. Set aside to cool.

5. Combine the ricotta and basil in a bowl.

6. Spread a little of the tomato over the base of a baking dish and arrange half the eggplant on top. Layer on the mushroom mixture, sweet potato, ricotta mixture, half the remaining tomato and then the remaining eggplant. Finish with the remaining tomato and sprinkle over the mozzarella. Bake for 35–45 minutes or until bubbling and golden. Serve with the baby spinach leaves.

Nutritional Information
(per serve)

Calories	**292**
Protein	**17.8 g**
Fat Total	**9.9 g**
Fat Saturated	**5.7 g**
Carbohydrates	**27.0 g**
Sugars	**15.6 g**
Sodium	**312.9 mg**
Dietary Fibre	**10.3 g**

Mish Tips

This is a great dish to use up leftover vegetables – zucchini, pumpkin and English spinach all work well here. You can also add some fresh herbs or a pinch of dried chilli flakes if you like.

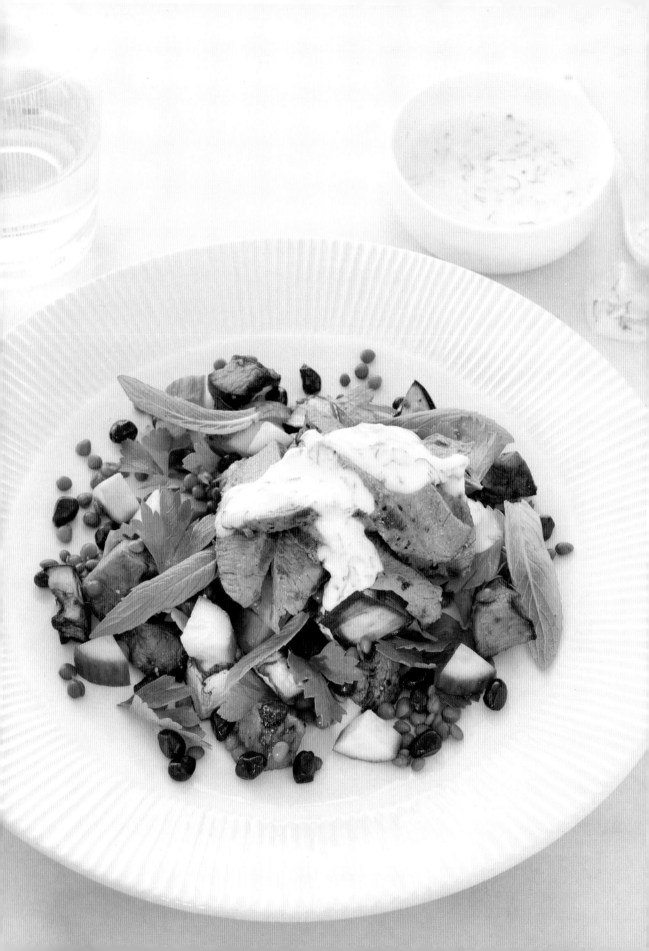

Warm lamb, pumpkin and pomegranate salad with minty yoghurt dressing

Pomegranate is packed with health benefits, and offers a refreshing tartness and crunch that is perfectly at home in this Middle Eastern-inspired lamb salad.

Serves: **2** · Prep time: **15 minutes** · Cooking time: **30 minutes** · Great for: *Weekend Lunch*

333 Calories   23.8 g Carbs

Ingredients

180 g peeled pumpkin, cut into
   2 cm pieces
1 eggplant, cut into 2 cm pieces
olive oil spray
3 tablespoons mint leaves
3 tablespoons low-fat natural yoghurt
1 clove garlic, crushed
200 g lamb loin fillet
65 g drained and rinsed tinned lentils
1 Lebanese cucumber, chopped
seeds of ½ pomegranate
½ cup flat-leaf parsley leaves

Method

1. Preheat the oven to 200°C (180°C fan-forced). Line a baking tray with baking paper.

2. Spread the pumpkin and eggplant over the prepared tray and lightly spray with olive oil. Bake for 30 minutes or until tender and lightly golden.

3. Meanwhile, finely chop half the mint leaves.

4. Combine the yoghurt, garlic, finely chopped mint and 1 tablespoon water in a small bowl. Season with freshly ground black pepper.

5. Heat a frying pan over medium–high heat. Lightly spray the lamb with olive oil and season with freshly ground black pepper. Add to the pan and cook for 4–5 minutes each side for medium, or until cooked to your liking. Transfer to a plate, cover loosely with foil and rest for 2 minutes, then finely slice.

6. Place the warm pumpkin and eggplant, lentils, cucumber, pomegranate seeds, parsley and the remaining mint in a large bowl. Season with freshly ground black pepper and gently toss to combine.

7. Divide the salad between two plates and top with the lamb. Drizzle with the minty yoghurt dressing and serve.

Nutritional Information

(per serve)

Calories	**333**
Protein	**36.9 g**
Fat Total	**6.7 g**
Fat Saturated	**2.0 g**
Carbohydrates	**23.8 g**
Sugars	**20.8 g**
Sodium	**219.0 mg**
Dietary Fibre	**11.9 g**

Less than 30 grams of carbs

Celeriac and white bean soup

With its attractive walnut and sage garnish, this delicious soup is an elegant lunch or dinner party dish.

Serves: **2** · Prep time: **20 minutes** · Cooking time: **50 minutes** · Great for: *Lunch, Dinner or Leftovers*

Ingredients

3 teaspoons olive oil

6 sage leaves

½ brown onion, finely chopped

1 clove garlic, crushed

400 g peeled celeriac, cut into
 1 cm pieces

2 cups salt-reduced vegetable stock

½ cup drained and rinsed tinned
 cannellini beans

½ cup low-fat milk

2 tablespoons walnuts, toasted and
 roughly chopped

Method

1. Heat the olive oil in a large saucepan over medium heat. Add the sage leaves and cook, tossing occasionally, for 2 minutes or until crisp. Remove with a slotted spoon and drain on paper towel. Add the onion and garlic to the pan and cook, stirring occasionally, for 3 minutes or until softened.

2. Add the celeriac, stock and 1 cup water. Cover and bring to the boil, then reduce the heat to medium–low and simmer for 40 minutes or until the celeriac is tender.

3. Stir in the cannellini beans and milk and set aside to cool slightly. Using a hand-held blender or food processor, blend until smooth, then return to the pan and gently reheat.

4. Ladle the soup into bowls and season with freshly ground black pepper. Sprinkle with the walnuts and crisp sage leaves and serve.

322 Calories	**21** g Carbs

Nutritional Information

(per serve)

Calories	**322**
Protein	**12.3 g**
Fat Total	**16.7 g**
Fat Saturated	**2.4 g**
Carbohydrates	**21.0 g**
Sugars	**14.7 g**
Sodium	**1135.3 mg**
Dietary Fibre	**14.9 g**

Mish Tips

Celeriac is a large knobbly root vegetable with pale yellow skin, white flesh and a distinctive flavour similar to celery. To peel it, you will need to use a knife to cut away the skin, rather than using a vegetable peeler. You can substitute the cannellini beans for other tinned beans, lentils or chickpeas if you like – just adjust the calories. To reduce the sodium content you can swap the stock for bone broth.

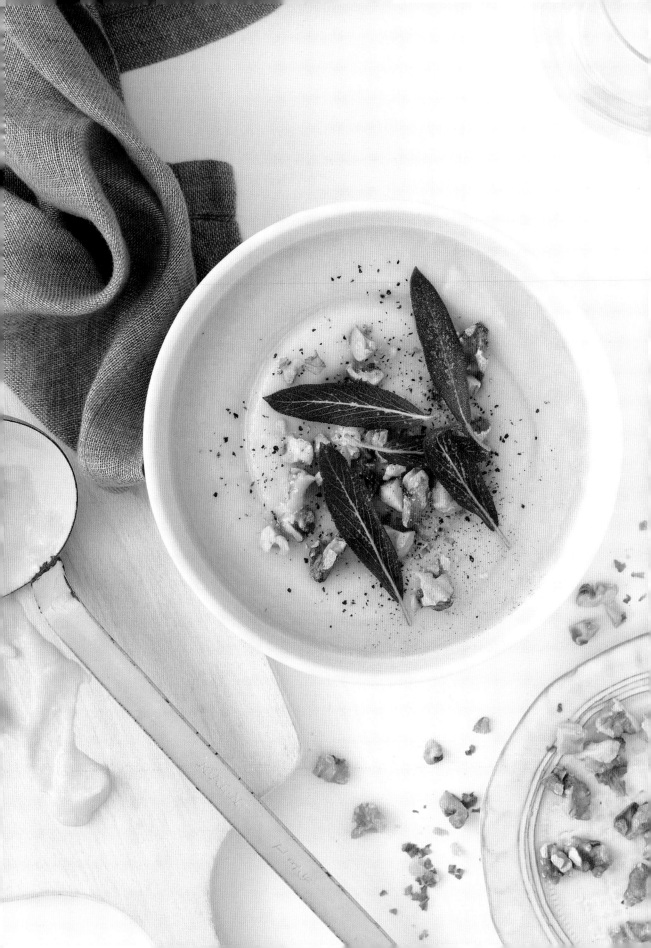

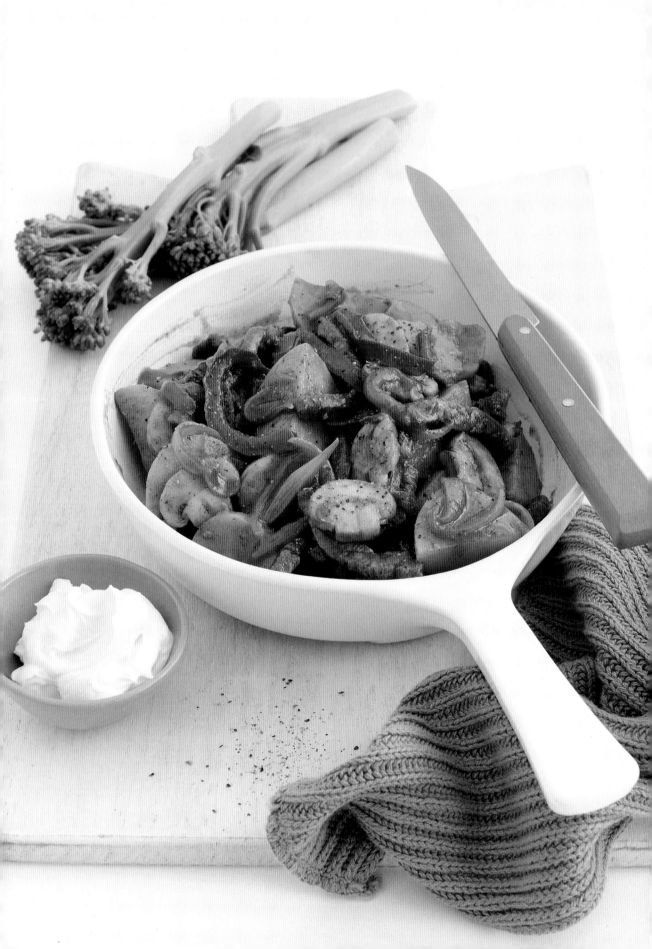

Veal goulash

I love herbs and spices, and the smoked paprika gives this dish its signature flavour. My version stays true to the traditional flavours but is lighter in calories, giving you the best of both worlds!

Serves: **2** • Prep time: **15 minutes** • Cooking time: **25 minutes** • Great for: *Lunch, Dinner or Leftovers*

333	20.3 g
Calories	Carbs

Ingredients

2 teaspoons olive oil

200 g veal schnitzel (no crumbs), cut into strips

½ brown onion, finely sliced

1 clove garlic, crushed

½ red capsicum, seeded and finely sliced

1 tablespoon tomato paste

½ teaspoon smoked paprika

¾ cup salt-reduced chicken stock

200 g baby potatoes, quartered

100 g mushrooms, sliced

1 bunch broccolini, trimmed

2 tablespoons extra light sour cream

Method

1. Heat half the olive oil in a large deep frying pan over medium–high heat. Add the veal and cook, stirring occasionally, for 3 minutes or until browned. Transfer to a plate. Heat the remaining oil in the pan, add the onion, garlic and capsicum and cook, stirring often, for 3 minutes or until softened.

2. Return the veal to the pan, then add the tomato paste and paprika and cook, stirring, for 1 minute. Add the stock and potato. Bring to the boil, then reduce the heat to medium–low and simmer, covered, for 12 minutes.

3. Add the mushroom. Cover and cook for a further 3 minutes or until the potato and mushroom are tender.

4. Meanwhile, cook the broccolini in a steamer set over a saucepan of simmering water for 3 minutes or until bright green and just tender.

5. Season the goulash with freshly ground black pepper and spoon into two bowls. Top with the sour cream and serve with the broccolini.

Nutritional Information
(per serve)

Calories	**333**
Protein	**35.5 g**
Fat Total	**10.5 g**
Fat Saturated	**3.3 g**
Carbohydrates	**20.3 g**
Sugars	**7.8 g**
Sodium	**385.5 mg**
Dietary Fibre	**7.2 g**

Mish Tips

Smoked paprika adds a mild smoky flavour to the goulash, but you can also use sweet paprika if that's what you have in your spice rack. If you have some fresh herbs handy, such as flat-leaf parsley, dill or chives, sprinkle them over before serving.

Roast beef dinner

Who doesn't love a roast? Simple to prepare and on the table in an hour. I'll say yes to that!

Serves: **2** · Prep time: **20 minutes** · Cooking time: **40 minutes** · Great for: *Weekend Lunch or Dinner*

279	22.2 g
Calories	Carbs

Ingredients

120 g brussels sprouts, trimmed
and halved

2 carrots, halved lengthways

140 g sweet potato, skin on, cut into
long wedges

85 g parsnip, halved lengthways

olive oil spray

1 teaspoon pure maple syrup

1 clove garlic, crushed

2 tablespoons finely chopped oregano

1 x 200 g lean beef fillet

Method

1. Preheat the oven to 190°C (170°C fan-forced). Line a large baking tray with baking paper.

2. Spread out the sprouts, carrot, sweet potato and parsnip on the prepared tray, lightly spray with olive oil and season with freshly ground black pepper. Drizzle over the maple syrup and roast for 40 minutes or until the vegetables are tender and golden.

3. Meanwhile, line a smaller baking tray with baking paper. Combine the garlic and oregano in a small bowl, then rub all over the beef fillet and season with freshly ground black pepper.

4. Lightly spray a small non-stick frying pan with olive oil and heat over medium heat. Add the fillet and brown all over. Transfer to the prepared small tray and roast for 20 minutes or until cooked to your liking. Remove to a board, cover loosely with foil and rest for a few minutes before slicing. Serve with the roast vegetables.

Nutritional Information
(per serve)

Calories	**279**
Protein	**27.0 g**
Fat Total	**7.3 g**
Fat Saturated	**2.5 g**
Carbohydrates	**22.2 g**
Sugars	**11.8 g**
Sodium	**113.8 mg**
Dietary Fibre	**10.0 g**

Mish Tips

Roast vegetables are simple and delicious! By all means, choose your own favourites for this recipe – try cauliflower and white or purple sweet potato.

Mexican cottage pie

This is such a favourite of mine — think chilli con carne with a sweet potato topping! If you don't have four individual baking dishes, just use one large dish and let everyone serve themselves at the table.

Serves: **4** · Prep time: **20 minutes** · Cooking time: **1 hour** · Great for: *Dinner*

Ingredients

olive oil spray

1 brown onion, finely chopped

2 cloves garlic, crushed

2 carrots, diced

1 zucchini, diced

1 celery stalk, diced

300 g lean beef mince

1 teaspoon ground cumin

pinch of chilli powder

1 x 400 g tin diced tomatoes

3 tablespoons roughly chopped coriander

500 g sweet potato, peeled and chopped

40 g parmesan, finely grated

Method

1. Lightly spray a large deep frying pan with olive oil and heat over medium heat. Add the onion and cook for 4 minutes or until softened. Stir in the garlic and cook for 30 seconds. Add the carrot, zucchini and celery and cook, stirring occasionally, for 5 minutes.

2. Increase the heat to medium–high. Add the mince and cook, breaking up the lumps with a wooden spoon, for 2 minutes or until lightly browned.

3. Add the cumin and chilli and cook for 30 seconds or until fragrant, then stir in the tomatoes and ¾ cup (180 ml) water. Cover and bring to the boil, reduce the heat to medium–low and simmer, stirring occasionally, for 20 minutes. Remove from the heat and stir in 2 tablespoons coriander.

4. Meanwhile, preheat the oven to 180°C (160°C fan-forced).

5. Cook the sweet potato in a steamer set over a saucepan of simmering water for 10 minutes or until tender. Roughly mash, then add the parmesan and stir to combine.

6. Spoon the beef mixture into four 1-cup capacity baking dishes. Spread the sweet potato mash over the top and lightly spray with olive oil. Bake for 30 minutes or until lightly browned. Sprinkle with the remaining coriander and serve.

311 **Calories** 24.8 g **Carbs**

Nutritional Information
(per serve)

Calories	**311**
Protein	**28.8 g**
Fat Total	**9.0 g**
Fat Saturated	**4.3 g**
Carbohydrates	**24.8 g**
Sugars	**13.8 g**
Sodium	**306.0 mg**
Dietary Fibre	**8.0 g**

Mish Tips

Double or even triple the ingredients to make a large batch of the beef mixture. Divide into portions and freeze in airtight containers. You may like to reserve some of the parmesan to scatter over the sweet potato just before baking.

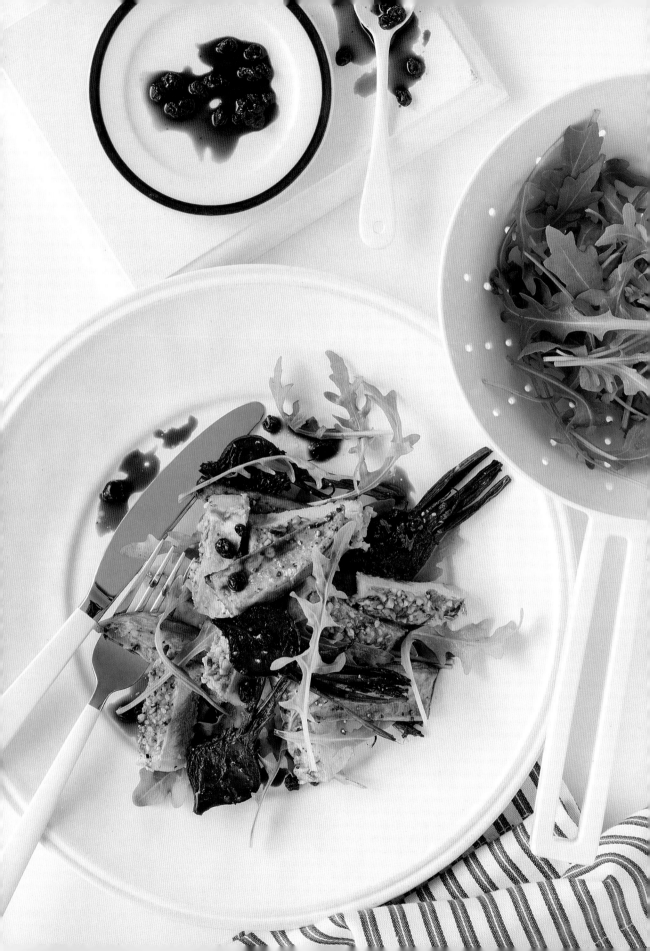

Dukkah-crusted pork with roasted vegetable salad

You will love the combination of flavours and textures in this warm salad.

Serves: **2** · Prep time: **15 minutes** · Cooking time: **35 minutes** · Great for: *Weekend Lunch*

Ingredients

10 g currants

1 teaspoon balsamic vinegar

175 g beetroot, chopped

200 g sweet potato, cut into wedges

olive oil spray

220 g lean pork steak, trimmed

1 tablespoon hummus

1 teaspoon dukkah

50 g baby rocket leaves

Method

1. Preheat the oven to 200°C (180°C fan-forced). Line a large baking tray with baking paper.

2. Combine the currants and balsamic vinegar in a small bowl and set aside.

3. Place the beetroot and sweet potato on the prepared tray. Lightly spray with olive oil and season with freshly ground black pepper. Roast for 30–35 minutes or until the vegetables are golden and tender.

4. Meanwhile, lightly spray a large non-stick frying pan with olive oil and heat over high heat. Add the pork and cook for 2 minutes each side or until golden. Transfer to a small baking tray. Spread the hummus over the pork, then sprinkle with the dukkah. Roast for 5 minutes.

5. Transfer the pork to a plate, cover loosely with foil and rest for 2 minutes, then thickly slice.

6. Place the roasted vegetables, pork and rocket on plates, add the balsamic currants and gently toss to combine. Season with freshly ground black pepper and serve.

289
Calories

25.7 g
Carbs

Nutritional Information

(per serve)

Calories	**289**
Protein	**31.9 g**
Fat Total	**5.1 g**
Fat Saturated	**0.7 g**
Carbohydrates	**25.7 g**
Sugars	**16.2 g**
Sodium	**144.0 mg**
Dietary Fibre	**7.5 g**

Mish Tips

Dukkah is an Egyptian spice mix of dried herbs, sesame seeds, nuts and spices. Look for it in the spice section of your supermarket. If you can't find it, use a blend of equal parts sesame seeds and ground cumin.

Less than 30 grams of carbs

Lamb steaks with spiced sweet potato and coriander mash

Lamb is an Aussie staple, and pairing it with such a swishy mash puts this dish on the world stage, I reckon!

Serves: **2** • Prep time: **15 minutes** • Cooking time: **15 minutes** • Great for: *Weekend Lunch or Dinner*

Ingredients

350 g peeled sweet potato, chopped

1 teaspoon olive oil

1 clove garlic, crushed

¼ teaspoon ground cumin

¼ teaspoon ground coriander

3 tablespoons chopped coriander

olive oil spray

200 g lean lamb steak

150 g broccolini, trimmed and cut into shorter lengths

Method

1. Place the sweet potato in a saucepan and cover with cold water. Bring to the boil and cook for 10 minutes or until tender. Drain well and set aside.

2. Wipe out the pan, add the olive oil and heat over medium heat. Add the garlic, cumin and ground coriander and cook, stirring, for 30 seconds or until aromatic. Add the sweet potato and mash until smooth. Stir in the fresh coriander and cover to keep warm.

3. Lightly spray a large non-stick frying pan with olive oil and heat over medium heat. Add the lamb and cook for 2 minutes each side for medium, or until cooked to your liking. Transfer to a plate, cover loosely with foil and rest for 2 minutes, then thickly slice.

4. Meanwhile, steam, boil or microwave the broccolini until tender. Drain.

5. Serve the lamb with the mash and broccolini, seasoned with freshly ground black pepper.

315	**25.4** g
Calories	Carbs

Nutritional Information

(per serve)

Calories	**315**
Protein	**28.7 g**
Fat Total	**9.4 g**
Fat Saturated	**2.5 g**
Carbohydrates	**25.4 g**
Sugars	**10.3 g**
Sodium	**98.0 mg**
Dietary Fibre	**8.5 g**

Mish Tips

You can use different spices each time you make this dish; it's great to mix it up. Ground turmeric paired with ground ginger is also amazing!

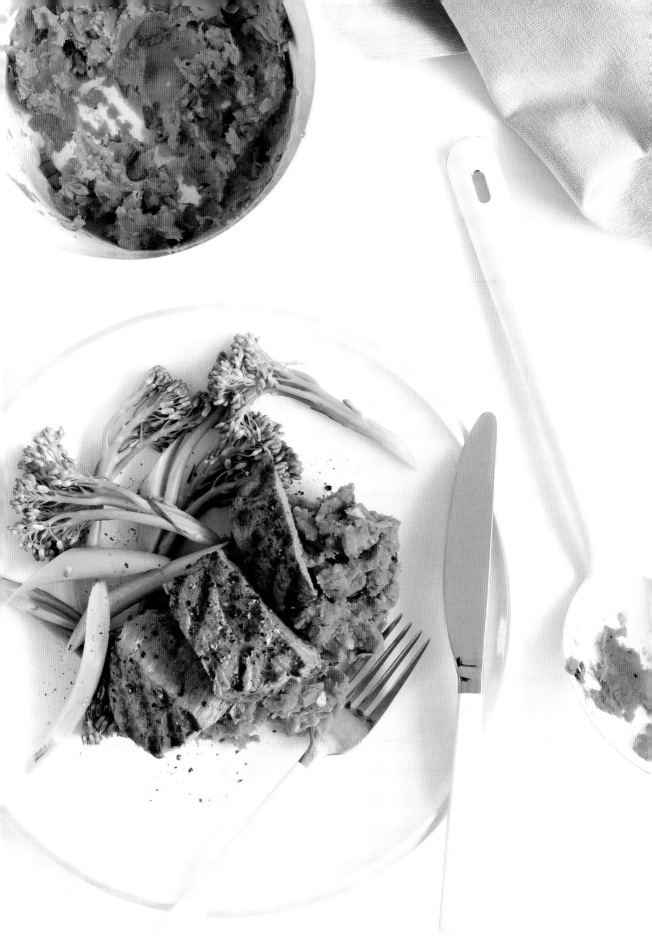

Smoked tofu, pickled ginger, avocado and quinoa *sushi*

This is a great family-friendly dish. Get the kids to roll their own sushi creations!

Serves: **2** · Prep time: **30 minutes** · Cooking time: **15 minutes** · Great for: *Lunch*

300	28.5 g
Calories	Carbs

Ingredients

⅓ cup white quinoa, rinsed and drained

2 sheets nori

100 g smoked tofu, cut into thin sticks

1 tablespoon pickled ginger, drained and chopped

¼ red capsicum, seeded and cut into thin sticks

1 Lebanese cucumber, cut into thin sticks

40 g avocado, finely sliced

1 tablespoon salt-reduced soy sauce

1 teaspoon wasabi paste

Method

1. Place the quinoa and 310 ml water in a small saucepan. Cover and bring to the boil, then reduce the heat to medium–low and simmer for 15 minutes or until the liquid has been absorbed. Transfer to a sieve and leave to drain and cool completely, fluffing occasionally with a fork to release the heat.

2. Lay one sheet of nori on a bamboo sushi mat. Spread half the cooled quinoa over one end (about one-third of the surface area). Arrange half the tofu, ginger, capsicum, cucumber and avocado in a line across the centre of the quinoa.

3. Using the mat, firmly roll up the nori to enclose the filling and dampen the end to seal. Repeat with the remaining nori and filling ingredients. Cut each roll into three pieces and serve straight away with the soy sauce and wasabi.

Nutritional Information
(per serve)

Calories	**300**
Protein	**17.5 g**
Fat Total	**11.9 g**
Fat Saturated	**2.0 g**
Carbohydrates	**28.5 g**
Sugars	**5.1 g**
Sodium	**920.3 mg**
Dietary Fibre	**4.9 g**

Mish Tips

Make sure the quinoa has cooled completely before spreading it over the nori. This recipe won't work with black quinoa as it is not as sticky as white quinoa. Trust me – I tried it!

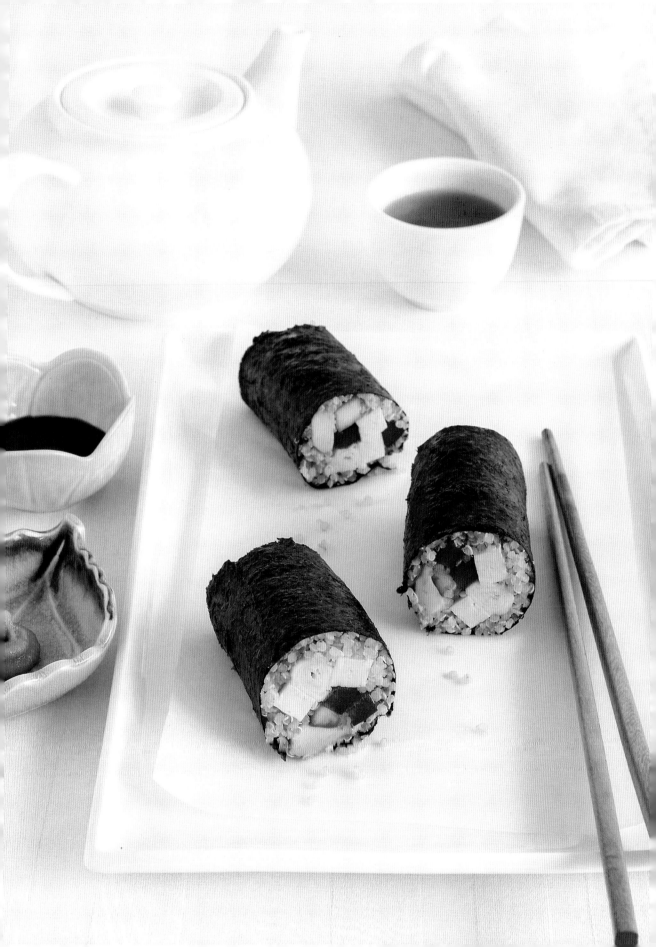

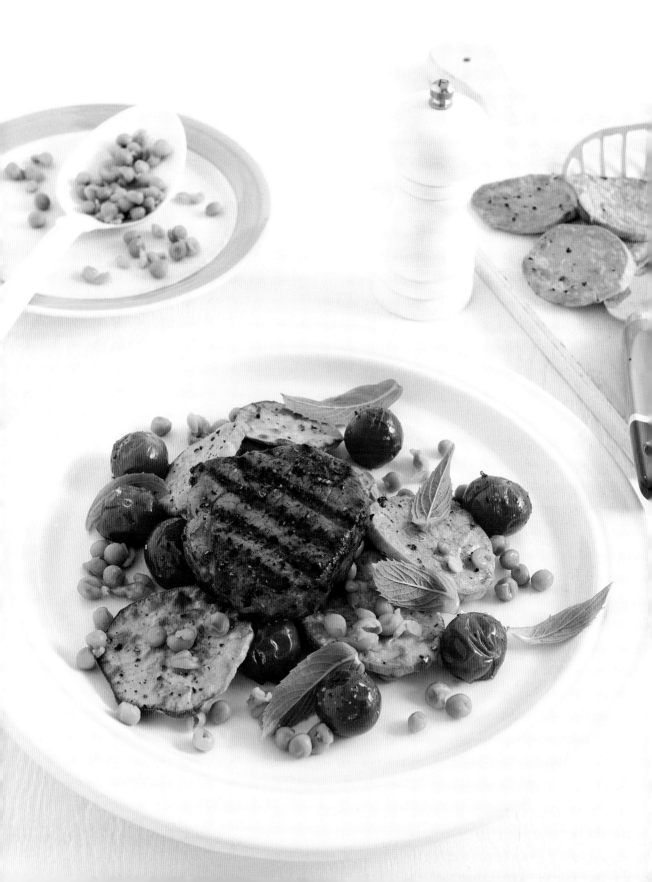

Peppered steak with mashed peas and roasted cherry tomatoes

Meat and three veg doesn't have to be boring! Hold back on the pepper if you're making this for little people.

Serves: **2** • Prep time: **15 minutes** • Cooking time: **25 minutes** • Great for: *Dinner*

Ingredients

300 g peeled sweet potato, cut into
    5 mm thick slices
olive oil spray
150 g cherry tomatoes
160 g frozen peas
2 x 100 g lean beef fillets
2 tablespoons mint leaves

Method

1. Preheat the oven to 200°C (180°C fan-forced). Line a large baking tray with baking paper.

2. Arrange the sweet potato in a single layer on the prepared tray and lightly spray with olive oil. Roast for 25 minutes or until tender.

3. Meanwhile, place the tomatoes in a small baking dish and roast for 15 minutes or until soft.

4. Cook the peas in a small saucepan of boiling water for 5 minutes or until just tender. Drain and crush slightly with a fork.

5. Heat a large non-stick frying pan over medium–high heat. Lightly spray both sides of the steaks with olive oil and season generously with freshly ground black pepper. Add to the pan and cook for 3 minutes each side for medium, or until cooked to your liking.

6. Divide the sweet potato, tomatoes, peas and steak between plates, sprinkle with mint and serve.

316	28 g
Calories	Carbs

Nutritional Information
(per serve)

Calories	**316**
Protein	**29.5 g**
Fat Total	**7.3 g**
Fat Saturated	**2.5 g**
Carbohydrates	**28.0 g**
Sugars	**12.1 g**
Sodium	**81.3 mg**
Dietary Fibre	**11.2 g**

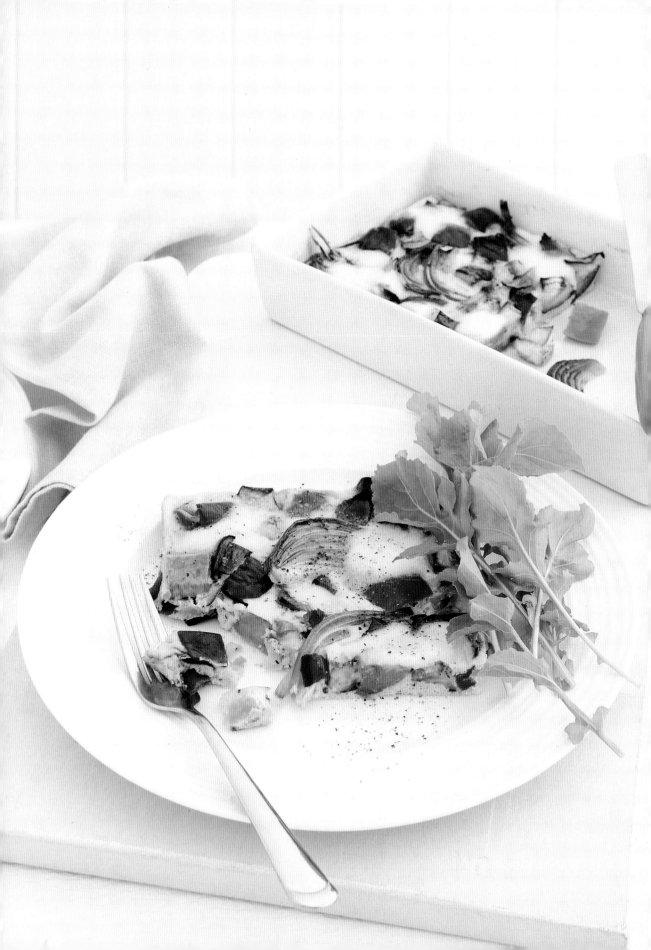

Roasted vegetable *frittata*

Making a frittata is a great way to use up your veggies, so nothing is wasted from your weekly shop!

Serves: **2** · Prep time: **20 minutes, plus 10 minutes cooling** · Cooking time: **55 minutes** ·
Great for: *Weekend Breakfast or Lunch*

Ingredients

325 g eggplant, chopped

1 red capsicum, seeded and chopped

125 g peeled sweet potato, chopped

½ red onion, cut into wedges

1 teaspoon olive oil

2 tablespoons chopped
    flat-leaf parsley

olive oil spray

3 cage-free eggs

½ cup low-fat milk

30 g bocconcini

25 g baby rocket leaves

Method

1. Preheat the oven to 200°C (180°C fan-forced). Line a baking tray with baking paper.

2. Place the eggplant, capsicum, sweet potato and onion on the prepared tray. Drizzle with the olive oil and toss to coat, then season with freshly ground black pepper. Roast for 25 minutes or until tender. Set aside to cool for 10 minutes, then mix in the parsley.

3. Reduce the oven temperature to 180°C (160°C fan-forced). Lightly spray a shallow 1.25 litre baking dish with olive oil. Spread the vegetables over the base of the dish. Whisk together the eggs and milk, and pour over the vegetables. Bake for 15 minutes.

4. Tear the bocconcini into pieces and scatter over the vegetable mixture. Bake for a further 10–15 minutes or until the frittata is set and lightly golden. Serve with the rocket leaves.

322	21.3 g
Calories	Carbs

Nutritional Information
(per serve)

Calories	**322**
Protein	**21.1 g**
Fat Total	**15.6 g**
Fat Saturated	**4.8 g**
Carbohydrates	**21.3 g**
Sugars	**15.9 g**
Sodium	**209.0 mg**
Dietary Fibre	**8.3 g**

Zucchini and herb *frittata*

Another version of my favourite egg staple, the frittata. You're getting how versatile this is, right?

Serves: **2** • Prep time: **15 minutes** • Cooking time: **30 minutes** • Great for: *Breakfast*

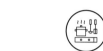

Ingredients

250 g potato, finely sliced

4 cage-free eggs

3 tablespoons low-fat milk

1 tablespoon chopped flat-leaf parsley

2 tablespoons chopped chives

olive oil spray

1 clove garlic, crushed

1 teaspoon finely grated lemon zest

1 zucchini, grated

125 g cherry tomatoes, halved

40 g low-fat feta, crumbled

20 g baby rocket leaves

Method

1. Place the potato in a microwave-safe bowl and add 2 tablespoons water. Cover and microwave on high for 2–3 minutes or until tender. Drain and set aside.

2. Place the eggs, milk, parsley and half the chives in a large bowl and whisk until well combined. Set aside.

3. Spray a 20 cm non-stick frying pan with olive oil and heat over high heat. Add the garlic and lemon zest and cook for 1 minute. Add the zucchini and cook for 2–3 minutes, then add the potato slices and scatter over the tomatoes.

4. Carefully pour the egg mixture into the pan and gently shake the pan to distribute it evenly. Crumble over the feta and sprinkle over the remaining chives. Reduce the heat to very low and cook for 5–10 minutes or until the frittata is set around the edges but still slightly runny in the centre. Preheat the grill to high.

5. Grill for 5–10 minutes or until the top is set, golden and puffed. Remove and rest for 5 minutes. Slide onto a large board, cut into wedges and serve topped with the rocket leaves.

336 Calories **20.9** g Carbs

Nutritional Information

(per serve)

Calories	**336**
Protein	**25.3 g**
Fat Total	**15.9 g**
Fat Saturated	**7.3 g**
Carbohydrates	**20.9 g**
Sugars	**5.4 g**
Sodium	**405.1 mg**
Dietary Fibre	**4.4 g**

Mish Tips

It is essential to use a non-stick frying pan for this frittata. Protect the handle of your pan with a damp tea towel while grilling. Take care as it will get hot. Frittata is delicious served warm or cold.

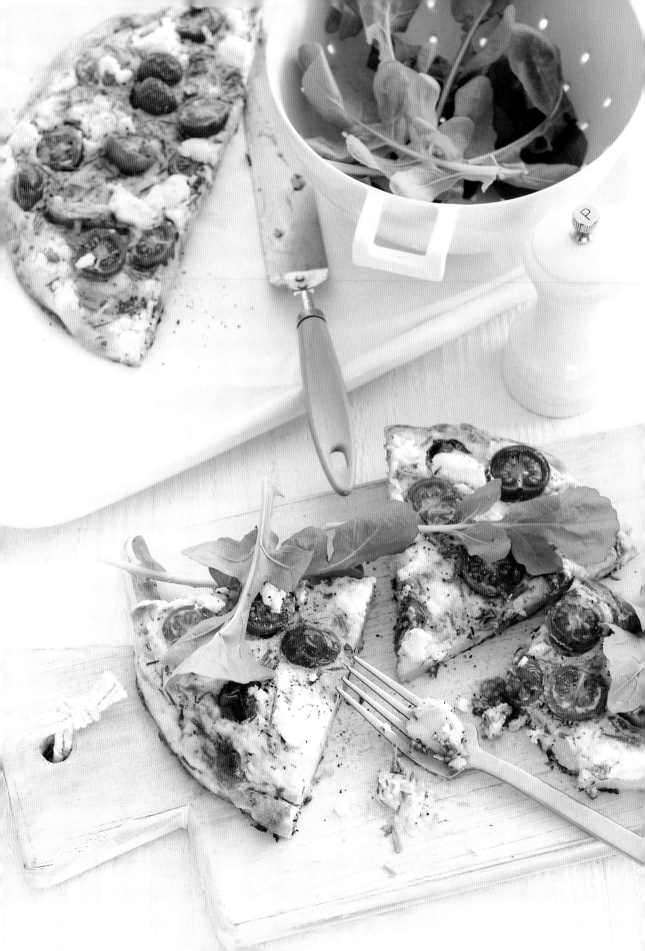

Charred chicken, corn and mango salad

As much as I love chicken, the real star of this dish is the corn — the charred flavour with the corn's natural sweetness is a delicious combination. The freshness of the mango rounds things out nicely.

Serves: **2** · Prep time: **20 minutes** · Cooking time: **10 minutes** · Great for: *Lunch*

298	25.1 g
Calories	Carbs

Ingredients

1 teaspoon dried oregano
pinch of smoked paprika
2 tablespoons lime juice
250 g lean chicken breast fillet
1 corn cob, husk and silks removed
4 spring onions, cut into 4 cm lengths
1 red capsicum, seeded and cut into thin strips
olive oil spray
50 g low-fat natural yoghurt
1 teaspoon wholegrain mustard
100 g baby spinach leaves
1 mango, sliced

Method

1. Rub the oregano, paprika and half the lime juice over the chicken. Lightly spray the chicken, corn, spring onion and capsicum with olive oil.

2. Heat a chargrill pan over medium heat or preheat a barbecue grill to medium. Add the chicken and corn and cook, turning occasionally, for 10 minutes or until the chicken is cooked through and the corn is nicely charred. Remove and set aside for a few minutes until the corn is cool enough to handle.

3. Meanwhile, add the spring onion and capsicum to the pan or barbecue and cook for 5 minutes or until lightly browned.

4. Combine the yoghurt, mustard and remaining lime juice to make a dressing.

5. Thinly slice the chicken. Use a sharp knife to cut down the length of the corn cob to remove the kernels.

6. Combine the corn, capsicum, spring onion, spinach and mango in a bowl. Divide between plates and top with the chicken. Drizzle over the yoghurt dressing and serve.

Nutritional Information

(per serve)

Calories	**298**
Protein	**36.0 g**
Fat Total	**4.6 g**
Fat Saturated	**0.9 g**
Carbohydrates	**25.1 g**
Sugars	**17.4 g**
Sodium	**174.7 mg**
Dietary Fibre	**7.8 g**

The easiest way to slice mango is to cut down both sides of the stone to remove the cheeks. Use a small sharp knife to score the flesh into thin slices, then simply peel away the skin.

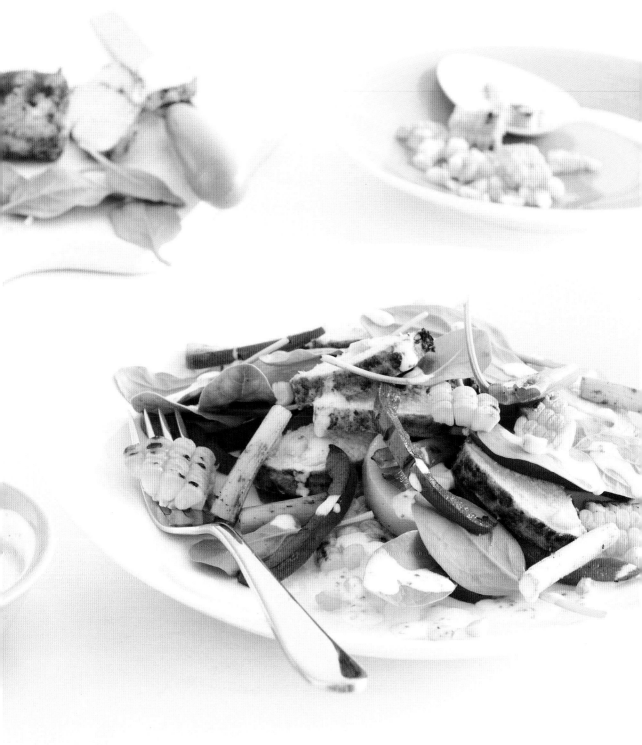

Tofu and greens stir-fry

This awesome Asian-style dish featuring tofu is bound to tempt all the vegetarians in the house!

Serves: **2** · Prep time: **10 minutes** · Cooking time: **15 minutes** · Great for: *Dinner*

Ingredients

70 g quinoa, rinsed and drained

1 teaspoon olive oil

150 g firm tofu, cut into 1 cm thick slices

200 g button mushrooms, halved

1 bunch Chinese broccoli (gai lan), chopped

60 g baby spinach leaves

100 g sugar snap peas, trimmed

1 tablespoon oyster sauce

2 spring onions, cut into 4 cm lengths

Method

1. Cook the quinoa in a saucepan of boiling water for 12 minutes. Drain well and fluff up the grains with a fork.

2. Meanwhile, heat the olive oil in a wok or large non-stick frying pan over medium–high heat. Add the tofu and cook for 1–2 minutes each side or until golden. Remove to a plate and set aside.

3. Add the mushroom and stir-fry for 2 minutes or until lightly golden. Transfer to the plate with the tofu. Add the Chinese broccoli, spinach and sugar snap peas to the wok, along with a splash of water to create steam, and stir-fry for 1–2 minutes. Add the oyster sauce and spring onion and stir-fry for 30 seconds.

4. Return the tofu and mushroom to the wok and toss to heat through (take care not to break up the tofu too much).

5. Divide the quinoa between bowls and top with the tofu, mushroom and greens.

331	**28.4** g
Calories	Carbs

Nutritional Information

(per serve)

Calories	**331**
Protein	**22.4 g**
Fat Total	**10.8 g**
Fat Saturated	**1.4 g**
Carbohydrates	**28.4 g**
Sugars	**3.9 g**
Sodium	**469.8 mg**
Dietary Fibre	**9.7 g**

Mish Tips

You can get packets of pre-cooked quinoa at the supermarket. You'll need 175 g cooked quinoa for this recipe.

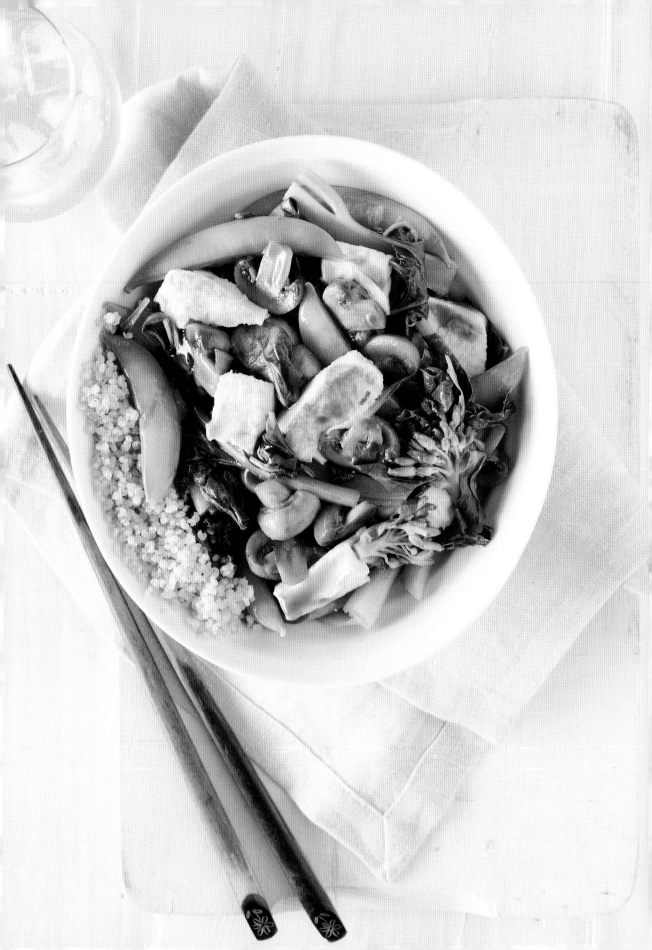

Summery lemon, honey and rosemary chicken

The rosemary really makes this dish. If you have it growing and the bush has long firm stems, you could strip off the leaves and use the stems as skewers.

Serves: **2** · Prep time: **20 minutes, plus 10 minutes chilling** · Cooking time: **15 minutes** · Great for: *Weekend Lunch*

305	24.1 g
Calories	Carbs

Ingredients

250 g lean chicken breast fillet, cut into thin strips

2 spring onions, cut into 4 cm lengths

2 lemons

2 teaspoons honey

1 tablespoon chopped rosemary

150 g potato, thickly sliced

200 g green beans, trimmed

olive oil spray

120 g baby rocket leaves

70 g low-fat natural yoghurt

1 teaspoon wholegrain mustard

Method

1. Thread the chicken and spring onion onto six skewers. Finely grate the zest of one lemon and squeeze the juice. Cut the remaining lemon into wedges and set aside. Combine the lemon zest and juice, honey and rosemary in a shallow dish. Add the chicken skewers and turn to coat, then cover and refrigerate for 10 minutes.

2. Cook the potato in a steamer set over a saucepan of simmering water for 12 minutes. Add the beans and cook for a further 3 minutes or until the beans are bright green and the potato is tender. Rinse the beans under cold running water to stop the cooking process and preserve the colour. Let the potato cool slightly.

3. Meanwhile, heat a chargrill pan over medium heat. Lightly spray the chicken skewers with olive oil, add to the pan and cook, turning regularly, for 10 minutes or until golden brown and cooked through.

4. Arrange the rocket, potato and beans on serving plates. Whisk together the yoghurt, mustard and 1 teaspoon water, and drizzle over the salad. Add the skewers to the plates and serve with the reserved lemon wedges.

Nutritional Information
(per serve)

Calories	**305**
Protein	**36.8 g**
Fat Total	**3.8 g**
Fat Saturated	**0.9 g**
Carbohydrates	**24.1 g**
Sugars	**12.5 g**
Sodium	**158.2 mg**
Dietary Fibre	**7.1 g**

Mish Tips

If you are using wooden or bamboo skewers, soak them in cold water for 15 minutes before threading the food on, to prevent them burning during cooking.

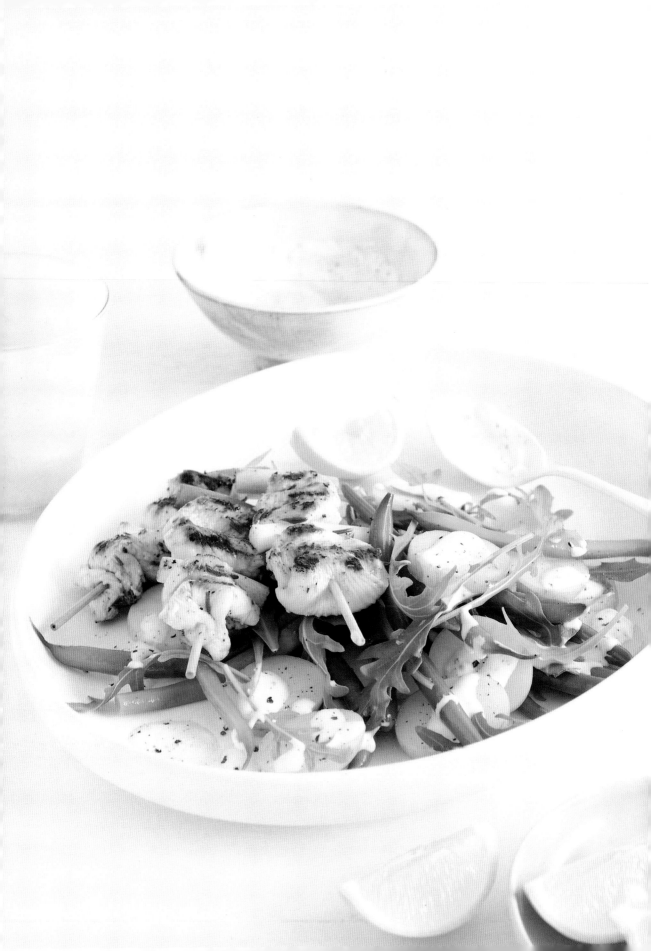

Beetroot salad with smoked tofu and beans

Tofu doesn't have to be plain in flavour. The smoked variety is delicious and really gives this salad a kick!

Serves: **2** • Prep time: **15 minutes** • Cooking time: **20 minutes** • Great for: *Weekend Lunch*

298	21.5 g
Calories	Carbs

Ingredients

240 g baby beetroot, stalks trimmed

50 g baby rocket leaves

1 cup bean sprouts, trimmed

½ cup drained and rinsed tinned cannellini beans

1 cage-free egg, hard-boiled, peeled and quartered

100 g smoked tofu, finely sliced

10 natural almonds, roughly chopped

1 tablespoon balsamic vinegar

1 tablespoon freshly squeezed orange juice

Method

1. Cook the beetroot in a large saucepan of boiling water for 15–20 minutes or until tender. Drain and cool.

2. Wearing prep gloves, peel the beetroot and cut in half lengthways.

3. Arrange the rocket leaves and bean sprouts on plates. Top with the beetroot, cannellini beans, egg, tofu and almonds. Whisk together the balsamic vinegar and orange juice and drizzle over the salad. Season with freshly ground black pepper and serve.

Nutritional Information
(per serve)

Calories	**298**
Protein	**21.6 g**
Fat Total	**11.9 g**
Fat Saturated	**1.8 g**
Carbohydrates	**21.5 g**
Sugars	**13.0 g**
Sodium	**648.1 mg**
Dietary Fibre	**10.6 g**

Mish Tips

If you have trouble finding smoked tofu, you can chargrill some sliced firm tofu to get a smoky flavour.

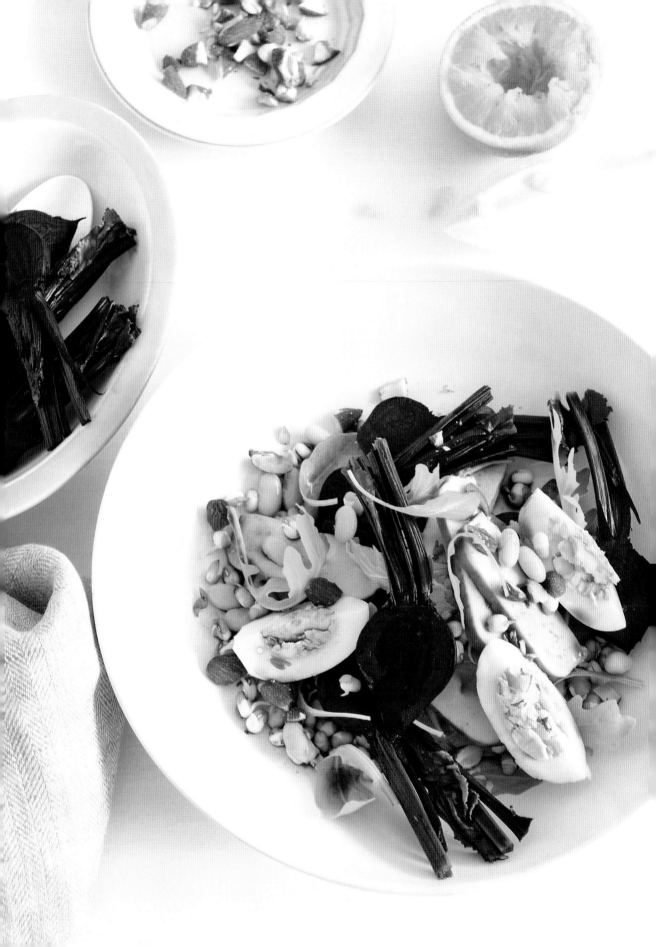

Pork with sweet potato chips and broccoli salad

Pork is so lean in fat and calories, it's not a meat that you should overlook. An average pork leg steak weighs 100 grams, so it's perfectly portion-controlled!

Serves: **2** · Prep time: **10 minutes** · Cooking time: **40 minutes** · Great for: *Dinner*

334	24.1 g
Calories	Carbs

Ingredients

100 g sweet potato, halved lengthways
   and sliced
olive oil spray
1 rindless bacon rasher, chopped
300 g broccoli, trimmed and cut
   into florets
30 g raisins
15 g flaked almonds
½ red onion, finely sliced
2 x 100 g lean pork steaks

Method

1. Preheat the oven to 200°C (180°C fan-forced). Line a baking tray with baking paper.

2. Place the sweet potato on the prepared tray and lightly spray with olive oil. Bake for 40 minutes or until tender.

3. Meanwhile, place the bacon in a small non-stick frying pan over medium heat and cook, stirring often, for 2–3 minutes or until lightly golden.

4. Cook the broccoli in a steamer set over a saucepan of simmering water for 3 minutes or until tender. Transfer to a large bowl and set aside to cool slightly.

5. Add the bacon, raisins, almonds and onion to the broccoli, season with freshly ground black pepper and toss to combine.

6. Heat a large non-stick frying pan over medium heat. Lightly spray both sides of the pork steaks with olive oil and season with freshly ground black pepper. Cook for 2 minutes each side for medium, or until cooked to your liking.

7. Divide the pork, sweet potato chips and broccoli salad between plates and serve.

Nutritional Information
(per serve)

Calories	**334**
Protein	**37.5 g**
Fat Total	**8.2 g**
Fat Saturated	**1.1 g**
Carbohydrates	**24.1 g**
Sugars	**16.9 g**
Sodium	**248.2 mg**
Dietary Fibre	**10.2 g**

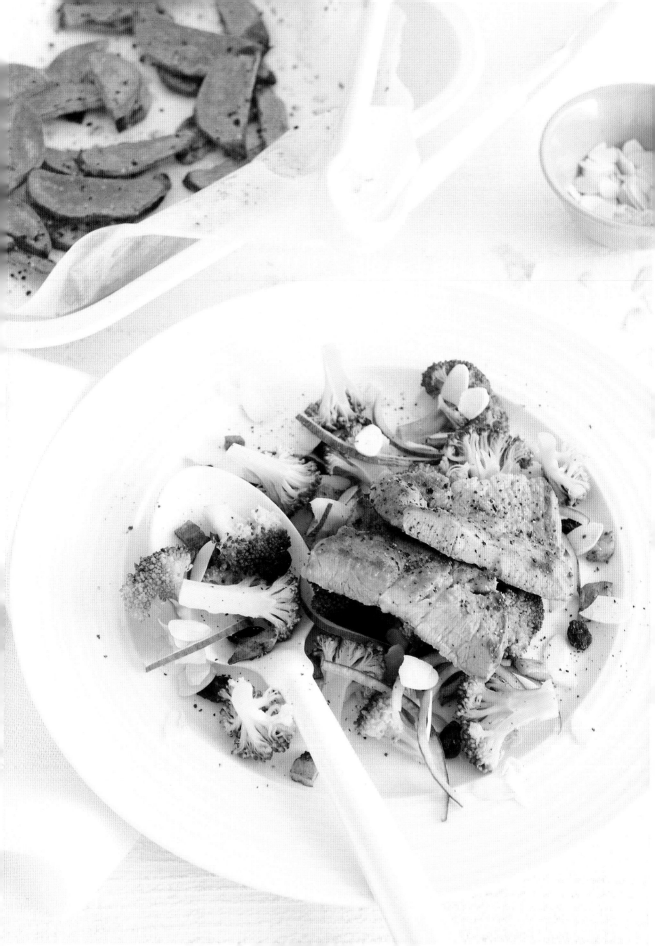

Raw broccoli and lentil salad

A great no-cook salad that's jam-packed with vegetable goodness.

Serves: **2** · Prep time: **15 minutes, plus 1 hour standing** · Great for: *Lunch*

Ingredients

300 g broccoli, trimmed and cut into small florets

2 tablespoons chopped flat-leaf parsley

1 tablespoon lemon juice

2 teaspoons olive oil

1 clove garlic, crushed

1 cup drained and rinsed tinned lentils

1 carrot, coarsely grated

1 tomato, chopped

2 tablespoons raisins

20 g flaked almonds

2 tablespoons low-fat natural yoghurt

Method

1. Combine the broccoli, parsley, lemon juice, olive oil and garlic in a large bowl. Cover and set aside for 1 hour to allow the flavours to infuse.

2. Add the lentils, carrot and tomato to the broccoli and season with freshly ground black pepper. Toss to combine, then divide between bowls and sprinkle with the raisins and almonds.

3. Stir 1 tablespoon water through the yoghurt and season with freshly ground black pepper. Serve on the side to drizzle over the salad.

294	23.9 g
Calories	Carbs

Nutritional Information

(per serve)

Calories	**294**
Protein	**16.8 g**
Fat Total	**12.6 g**
Fat Saturated	**1.2 g**
Carbohydrates	**23.9 g**
Sugars	**14.4 g**
Sodium	**356.7 mg**
Dietary Fibre	**9.6 g**

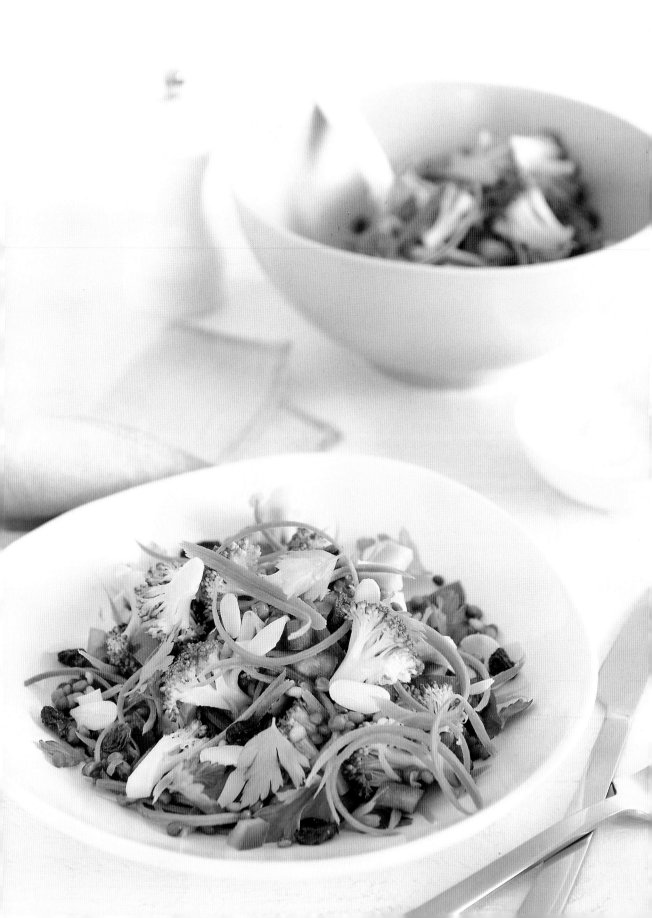

Sweet potato, mushroom and feta stacks

This elegant vegetarian recipe is a fancy way to dress up humble veggies. It's easy to prepare, so it's a great one for entertaining.

Serves: **4** · Prep time: **20 minutes** · Cooking time: **25 minutes** · Great for: *Dinner*

Ingredients

400 g sweet potato, peeled and
    roughly chopped
30 g extra light sour cream
olive oil spray
400 g eggplant, cut into 1 cm
    thick rounds
4 field mushrooms, stems removed
200 g low-fat feta, cut into 1 cm cubes
80 g baby rocket leaves

Method

1. Cook the sweet potato in a steamer set over a saucepan of simmering water until tender. Drain, then mash the sweet potato with the sour cream until smooth.

2. Meanwhile, lightly spray a chargrill pan with olive oil and heat over medium–high heat. Add the eggplant, in batches if necessary, and cook for 3–4 minutes each side or until tender and lightly golden.

3. Preheat the grill to medium–high. Place the mushrooms, stem side up, on a baking tray and grill for 5 minutes or until tender. Top with the feta and grill until golden.

4. Divide the sweet potato mash among plates. Top with the eggplant slices, mushrooms and rocket. Season with freshly ground black pepper and serve.

262 Calories   23.5 g Carbs

Nutritional Information
(per serve)

Calories	**262**
Protein	**20.3 g**
Fat Total	**9.0 g**
Fat Saturated	**10.0 g**
Carbohydrates	**23.5 g**
Sugars	**11.3 g**
Sodium	**583.6 mg**
Dietary Fibre	**7.9 g**

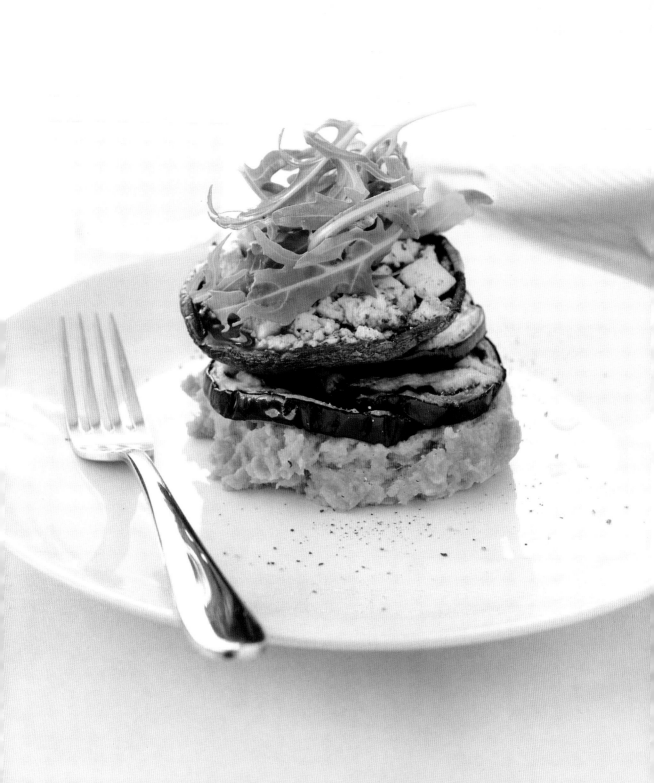

Beef and bean soup

I love soups. They are so warming and filling, and this one is full of delicious goodness. It comes together really quickly too.

Serves: **2** · Prep time: **10 minutes** · Cooking time: **10 minutes** · Great for: *Lunch, Dinner or Leftovers*

Ingredients

2 teaspoons olive oil

1 brown onion, chopped

1 zucchini, chopped

1 carrot, grated

1 teaspoon sweet paprika

1 x 400 g tin diced tomatoes

1½ cups salt-reduced beef stock

150 g lean beef fillet, finely sliced

3 tablespoons drained and rinsed tinned red kidney beans

Method

1. Heat the olive oil in a large saucepan over medium–high heat. Add the onion, zucchini and carrot, and cook, stirring, for 2 minutes. Add the paprika and cook, stirring, for 1 minute.

2. Add the tomatoes and stock. Bring to the boil, then reduce the heat to medium and cook for 3 minutes. Stir in the beef and kidney beans and simmer for 2 minutes or until the beef is just cooked through and the vegetables are tender. Ladle into bowls, season with freshly ground black pepper and serve.

288	**21** g
Calories	Carbs

Nutritional Information
(per serve)

Calories	**288**
Protein	**24.0 g**
Fat Total	**10.6 g**
Fat Saturated	**2.8 g**
Carbohydrates	**21.0 g**
Sugars	**13.6 g**
Sodium	**705.7 mg**
Dietary Fibre	**8.5 g**

Mish Tips

If you don't have any liquid stock to hand, you can use ½ teaspoon stock powder dissolved in 1½ cups boiling water instead. Use smoked paprika for a slightly different flavour if you like.

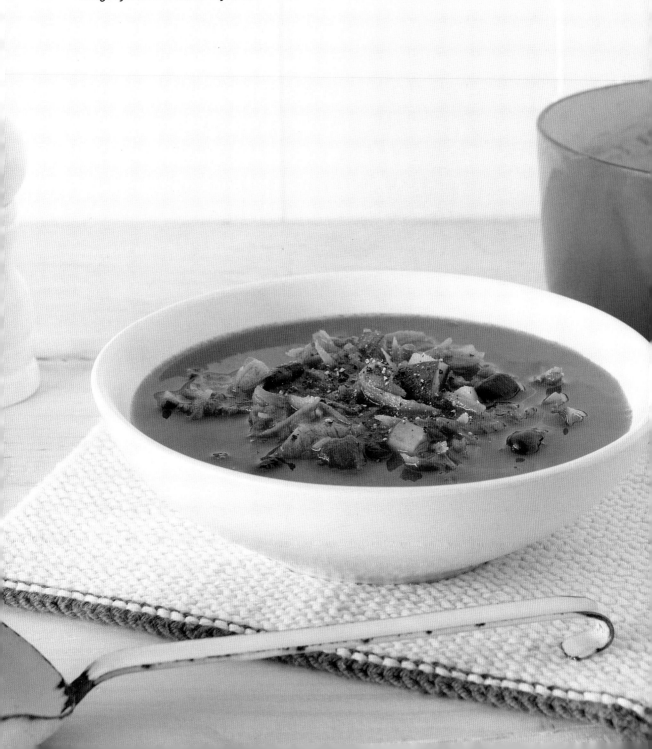

> **MORE THAN**

30

grams of carbs

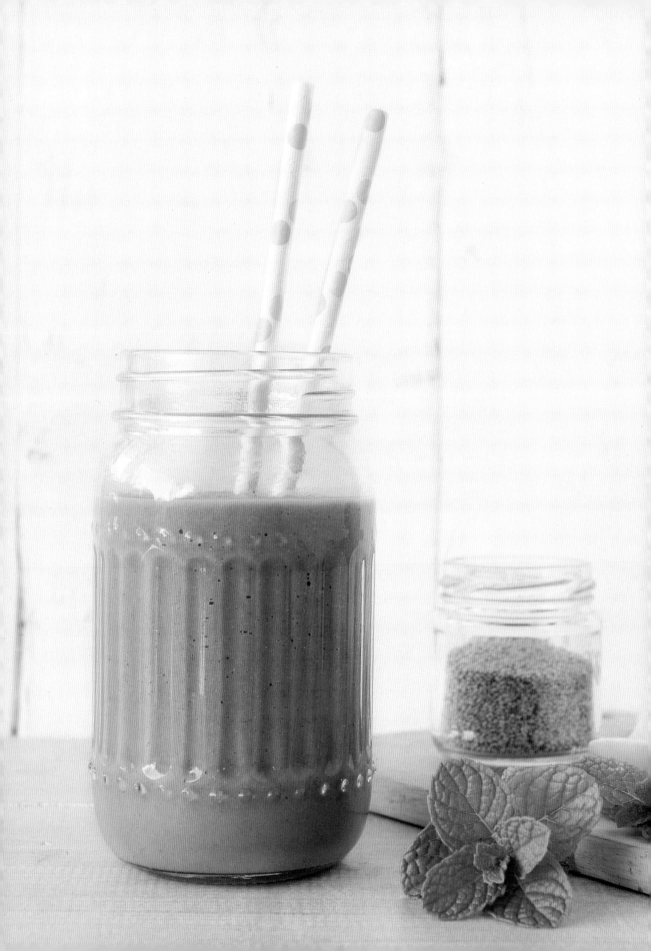

Super green smoothie

I start every day with a super green smoothie and this is one of my favourite recipes.

Serves: **2** · Prep time: **10 minutes** · Great for: *Breakfast*

Ingredients

120 g avocado, flesh scooped

240 g pineapple, chopped and frozen

1 banana, chopped and frozen

80 g baby spinach leaves

3 teaspoons chia seeds

2 tablespoons chopped mint

1½ cups coconut water

Method

1. Place all the ingredients in a blender and blend until smooth. Pour into two glasses and serve.

306	30.5 g
Calories	Carbs

Nutritional Information

(per serve)

Calories	**306**
Protein	**6.2 g**
Fat Total	**16.8 g**
Fat Saturated	**3.4 g**
Carbohydrates	**30.5 g**
Sugars	**25.8 g**
Sodium	**70.9 mg**
Dietary Fibre	**8.1 g**

Prepare the fruit ahead of time and freeze in zip-lock bags for a quick and easy breakfast.

Summer smoothie bowl

This breakfast is as pretty to look at as it is quick and easy to make.

Serves: **2** • Prep time: **5 minutes** • Great for: *Breakfast*

Ingredients

1 mango, chopped and frozen

1 banana, chopped and frozen

1½ cups low-fat natural yoghurt

1 passionfruit, halved, seeds and
   juice scraped

1 tablespoon desiccated
   coconut, toasted

3 teaspoons pumpkin seeds

1 tablespoon flaked almonds

Method

1. Place the mango, banana and yoghurt in a food processor and process until smooth. Divide between two bowls.

2. Top with the passionfruit pulp, coconut, pumpkin seeds and almonds and serve.

276	31.5 g
Calories	Carbs

Nutritional Information
(per serve)

Calories	**276**
Protein	**15.9 g**
Fat Total	**7.5 g**
Fat Saturated	**2.8 g**
Carbohydrates	**31.5 g**
Sugars	**27.3 g**
Sodium	**155.4 mg**
Dietary Fibre	**6.1 g**

Buy fruit when it is cheap and in season and freeze in zip-lock bags for a quick breakfast.

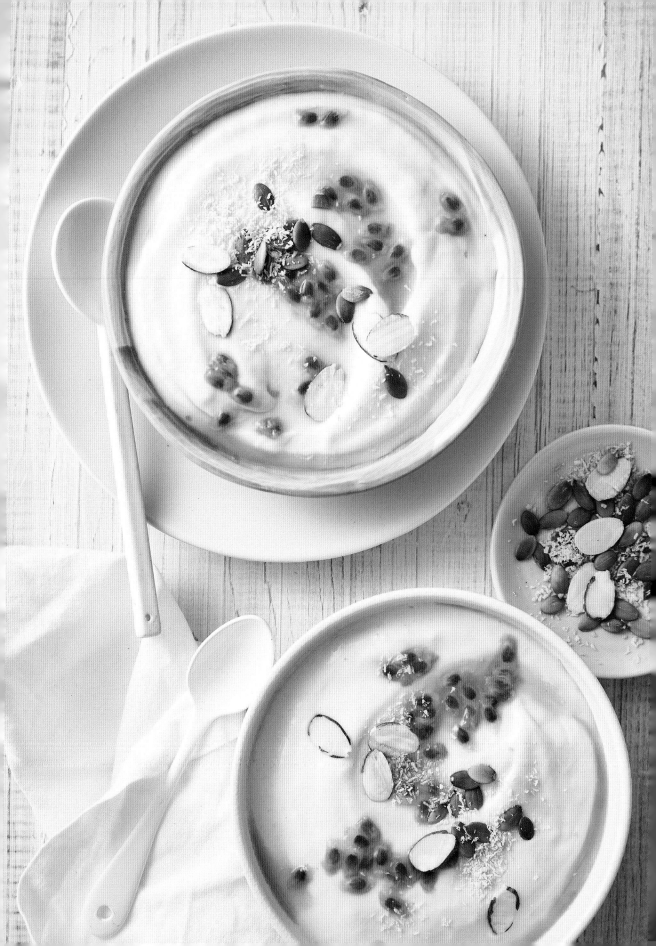

Tropical fruit salad with toasted coconut yoghurt

There's nothing boring about fruit salad when you add a tropical twist and a good dollop of coconut yoghurt. This is so good it could double as dessert!

Serves: **1** · Prep time: **10 minutes** · Cooking time: **5 minutes** · Great for: *Breakfast*

315	44 g
Calories	Carbs

Ingredients

2 tablespoons shredded coconut

300 g peeled pineapple, chopped

200 g peeled papaya or pawpaw, chopped

2 mango cheeks, flesh chopped

10 mint leaves

1 passionfruit, halved, seeds and juice scraped

⅓ cup low-fat Greek-style yoghurt

Method

1. Place the coconut in a small frying pan over medium heat and cook, stirring often, for 2 minutes or until lightly toasted. Transfer to a plate and set aside to cool.

2. Gently toss together the pineapple, papaya or pawpaw, mango and mint in a large bowl. Spoon the passionfruit pulp over the top.

3. Place the yoghurt and three-quarters of the coconut in a small bowl and stir to combine.

4. Spoon the coconut yoghurt over the fruit, sprinkle with the remaining coconut and serve.

Nutritional Information

(per serve)

Calories	**315**
Protein	**6.5 g**
Fat Total	**10.0 g**
Fat Saturated	**7.7 g**
Carbohydrates	**44.0 g**
Sugars	**42.1 g**
Sodium	**48.0 mg**
Dietary Fibre	**13.8 g**

Mish Tips

Red papaya is oval shaped with deep-orange flesh and has a much milder flavour than the larger yellow-fleshed pawpaw. Either is fine here, or replace it with any other tropical fruit. Strawberries would work a treat too.

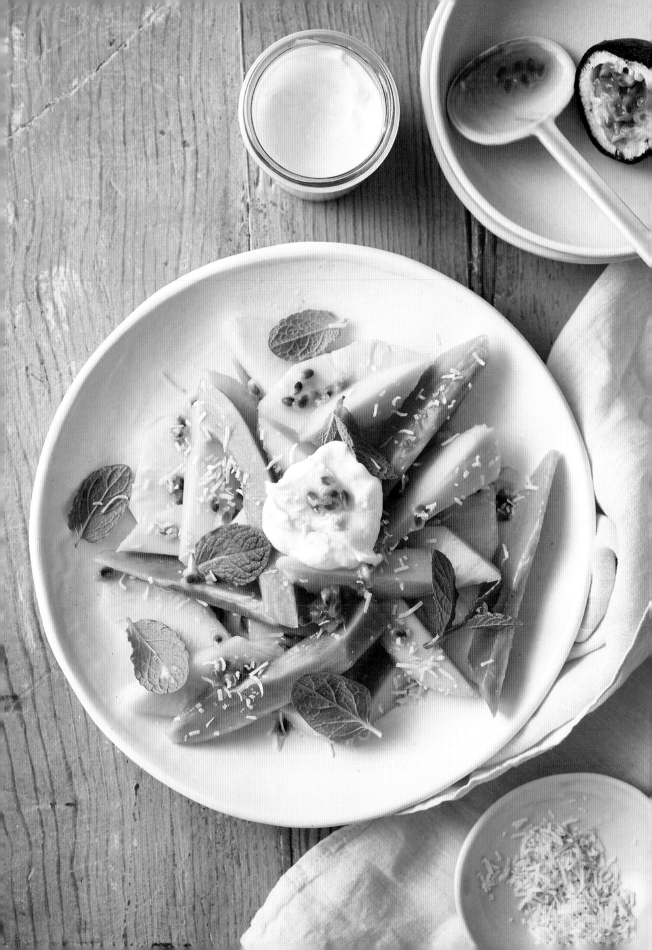

Buddha bowl

Who needs to go to a hipster cafe when you can make this at home for half the price? Fresh, delicious and so good for you.

Serves: **2** · Prep time: **15 minutes** · Cooking time: **25 minutes** · Great for: *Weekend Breakfast or Lunch*

Ingredients

250 g peeled pumpkin, cut into
   2 cm pieces

½ teaspoon ground turmeric

olive oil spray

350 g cauliflower, cut into florets

3 tablespoons red quinoa, rinsed
   and drained

40 g kale, stalks removed, leaves torn

2 tablespoons lemon juice

50 g low-fat natural yoghurt

2 teaspoons tahini

120 g beetroot, coarsely grated

2 teaspoons pumpkin seeds

Method

1. Preheat the oven to 200°C (180°C fan-forced). Line a baking tray with baking paper.

2. Arrange the pumpkin on the prepared tray, sprinkle with half the turmeric and lightly spray with olive oil. Roast for 10 minutes. Add the cauliflower to the tray, sprinkle with the remaining turmeric and lightly spray with olive oil. Roast for a further 15 minutes or until the vegetables are tender and lightly browned.

3. Meanwhile, cook the quinoa in a saucepan of boiling water for 12 minutes. Drain well and fluff up the grains with a fork.

4. Place the kale in a large bowl and drizzle with 1 tablespoon lemon juice. Massage the juice into the leaves for a minute until they are soft and slightly wilted. Combine the remaining lemon juice with the yoghurt and tahini and whisk until smooth.

5. Arrange the roasted vegetables, quinoa, kale and beetroot in two bowls. Drizzle with the dressing and season with freshly ground black pepper. Sprinkle the pumpkin seeds over the top and serve.

330	35.9 g
Calories	Carbs

Nutritional Information
(per serve)

Calories	**330**
Protein	**14.8 g**
Fat Total	**10.5 g**
Fat Saturated	**1.3 g**
Carbohydrates	**35.9 g**
Sugars	**18.9 g**
Sodium	**124.8 mg**
Dietary Fibre	**13.5 g**

Mish Tips

We used red quinoa but you can use white if you like. Use prep gloves to grate the beetroot to avoid staining your hands.

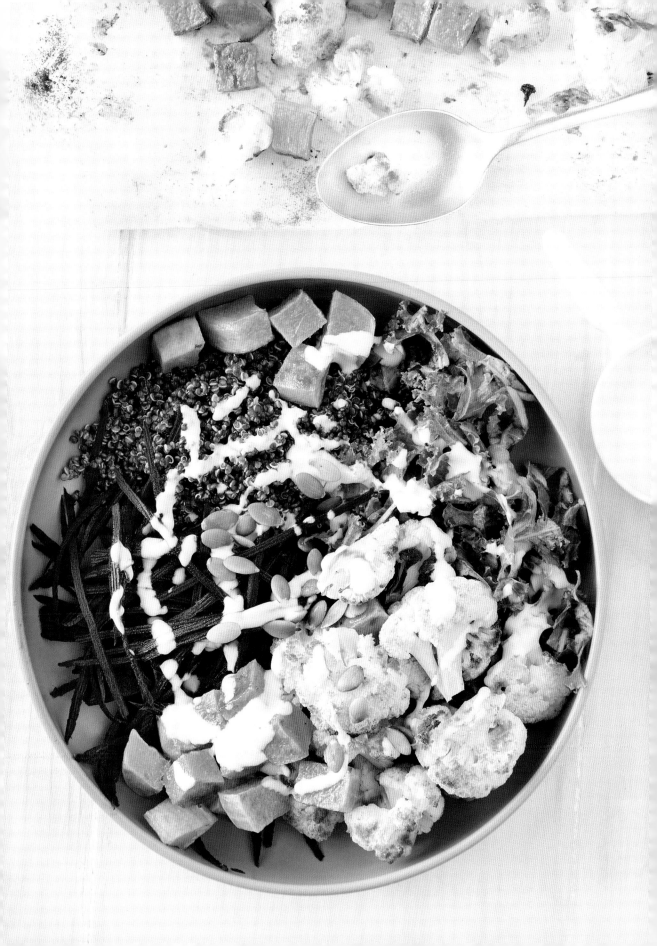

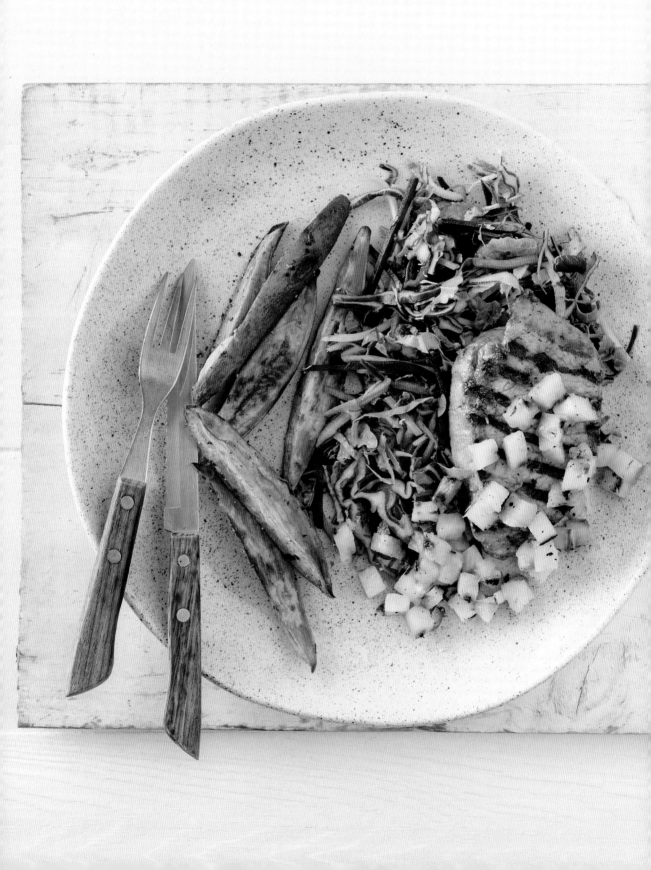

Pork with grilled pineapple

Pork, pineapple and ginger is a flavour combination that everyone in the family will love. Add caramelised sweet potato wedges and you're onto a winner!

Serves: **4** · Prep time: **15 minutes, plus 20 minutes marinating** · Cooking time: **30 minutes** · Great for: *Dinner*

317 Calories **31** g Carbs

Ingredients

500 g small sweet potatoes, each cut lengthways into 6 wedges
olive oil spray
4 x 125 g lean pork steaks
2 teaspoons finely grated ginger
1 tablespoon salt-reduced soy sauce
250 g pineapple, peeled and cut into 4 slices
200 g dry coleslaw mix
2 tablespoons lime juice

Method

1. Preheat the oven to 200°C (180°C fan-forced). Line a baking tray with baking paper.

2. Place the sweet potato wedges on the prepared tray and lightly spray with olive oil. Roast for 30 minutes or until tender and caramelised.

3. Meanwhile, toss the pork with the ginger and soy sauce. Cover and marinate in the fridge for about 20 minutes.

4. Heat a barbecue, chargrill or frying pan over medium–high heat. Lightly spray the pork with olive oil and cook for 3 minutes each side. Remove to a plate and cover to keep warm. Cook the pineapple for 1–2 minutes each side or until nicely golden. Cool slightly, then dice the pineapple, discarding the core.

5. Toss the coleslaw mix with the lime juice. Serve with the pork, pineapple and sweet potato wedges.

Nutritional Information
(per serve)

Calories	**317**
Protein	**34.5 g**
Fat Total	**4.9 g**
Fat Saturated	**1.0 g**
Carbohydrates	**31.0 g**
Sugars	**20.1 g**
Sodium	**373.5 mg**
Dietary Fibre	**5.0 g**

Mish Tips

To make the wedges, we used very small sweet potatoes, which you can find in some supermarkets. Otherwise just cut a larger sweet potato into slices or chip shapes.

Quinoa and kidney bean chilli

This is so hearty and filling, you would never guess it's so low in calories!

Serves: **2** • Prep time: **15 minutes** • Cooking time: **20 minutes** • Great for: *Lunch, Dinner or Leftovers*

299	35.1 g
Calories	Carbs

Ingredients

3 teaspoons olive oil

½ brown onion, finely chopped

1 clove garlic, crushed

1 celery stalk, chopped

½ red capsicum, seeded and chopped

1 x 400 g tin diced tomatoes

1 zucchini, chopped

pinch of cayenne pepper

3 tablespoons quinoa, rinsed and drained

½ cup drained and rinsed tinned red kidney beans

3 tablespoons chopped coriander

⅓ cup low-fat natural yoghurt

Method

1. Heat the olive oil in a saucepan over medium heat. Add the onion, garlic, celery and capsicum and cook, stirring, for 3 minutes or until softened.

2. Add the tomatoes, zucchini, cayenne pepper and quinoa. Bring to the boil, then reduce the heat to medium–low and simmer, covered, for 15 minutes or until the quinoa is tender. Remove from the heat and stir in the beans and coriander. Season with freshly ground black pepper.

3. Divide the chilli mixture between two bowls, top with the yoghurt and serve.

Nutritional Information
(per serve)

Calories	**299**
Protein	**12.4 g**
Fat Total	**9.9 g**
Fat Saturated	**1.4 g**
Carbohydrates	**35.1 g**
Sugars	**13.9 g**
Sodium	**352.1 mg**
Dietary Fibre	**10.1 g**

Don't forget to rinse the quinoa, otherwise it will have a bitter taste. You can swap the kidney beans for other tinned beans, lentils or chickpeas if you like — just adjust the calories.

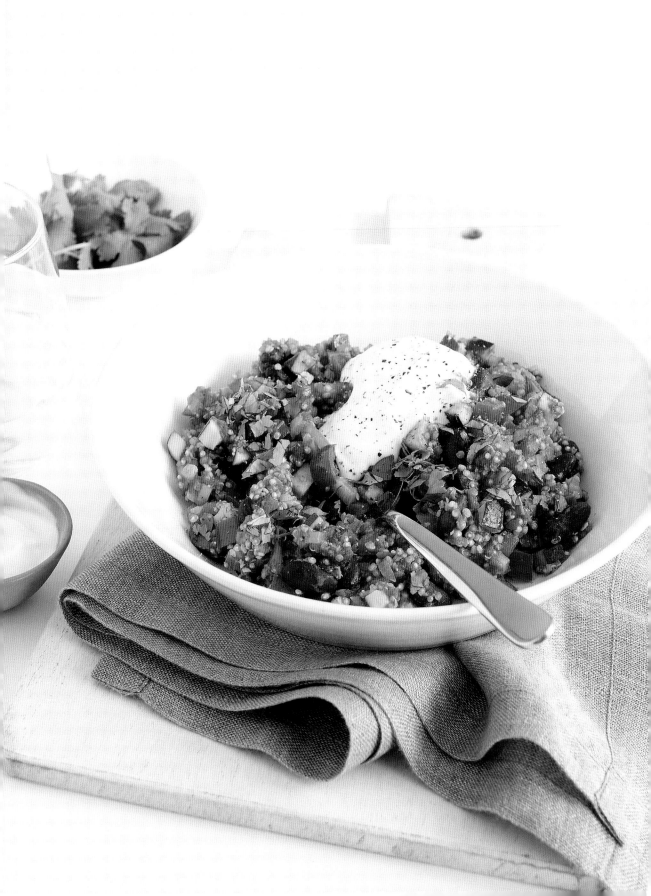

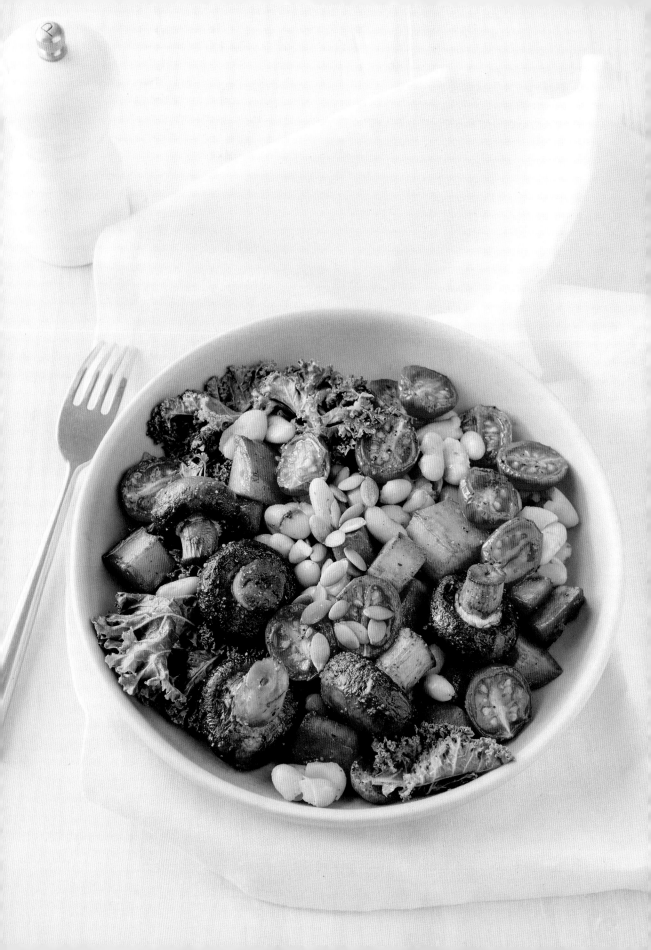

Roasted mushrooms with honey soy sweet potato

Mushrooms are filling and nutritious, and combined with the cannellini beans they make a really satisfying vego meal.

Serves: **2** · Prep time: **15 minutes** · Cooking time: **30 minutes** · Great for: *Dinner*

Ingredients

200 g sweet potato, peeled and cut into 3 cm pieces
1 tablespoon salt-reduced soy sauce
1 clove garlic, crushed
1 teaspoon honey
2 teaspoons sesame oil
200 g button mushrooms
200 g cherry tomatoes, halved
1 x 400 g tin cannellini beans, drained and rinsed
olive oil spray
60 g kale, stalks removed, leaves roughly chopped
2 teaspoons pumpkin seeds

Method

1. Preheat the oven to 200°C (180°C fan-forced). Line two large baking trays with baking paper.

2. Place the sweet potato, soy sauce, garlic, honey and sesame oil in a large bowl and toss to coat. Spread over one of the prepared trays and roast for 30 minutes or until tender and golden.

3. Meanwhile, spread the mushrooms, tomatoes and cannellini beans over the remaining tray. Season with freshly ground black pepper and lightly spray with olive oil, then roast for 20 minutes or until soft.

4. Meanwhile, lightly spray a large non-stick frying pan with olive oil and heat over medium–high heat. Add the kale and cook, stirring, for 1–2 minutes or until wilted, adding a splash of water to create steam.

5. Divide the sweet potato, mushrooms, tomatoes, beans and kale between two plates. Sprinkle with the pumpkin seeds and serve.

312	**35.5** g
Calories	Carbs

Nutritional Information
(per serve)

Calories	**312**
Protein	**15.2 g**
Fat Total	**8.6 g**
Fat Saturated	**1.4 g**
Carbohydrates	**35.5 g**
Sugars	**14.4 g**
Sodium	**686.8 mg**
Dietary Fibre	**14.7 g**

Warm winter vegetable salad

That's right, salads aren't just for summer. Here we roast the veggies to enhance their natural sweetness, and add beans for protein and fresh thyme to liven things up!

Serves: **2** • Prep time: **15 minutes** • Cooking time: **45 minutes** • Great for: *Weekend Lunch or Dinner*

Ingredients

200 g beetroot, trimmed and scrubbed
200 g sweet potato, cut into thick chips
olive oil spray
1 teaspoon sweet paprika
1 red onion, cut into 8 wedges
200 g brussels sprouts, trimmed
 and halved
200 g cauliflower, cut into florets
2 cloves garlic, unpeeled
2 teaspoons red wine vinegar
2 teaspoons olive oil
½ cup drained and rinsed tinned
 borlotti beans
2 teaspoons thyme leaves

We used 4 baby beetroots (to a total of 200 g), evenly sized so they cook at the same time. Larger beetroot will need longer in the oven. If some veggies are ready before the others, take them off the tray and keep warm on a plate while the others finish cooking. You can use any type of paprika in this recipe. Just use what you have in your pantry — it won't change the carbohydrate or calorie levels.

Method

1. Preheat the oven to 190°C (170°C fan-forced).

2. Wrap the beetroot in foil and place on a small baking tray. Roast for 45 minutes or until tender when pierced with a small knife. Cool, then, wearing prep gloves, slip off the skins and cut into wedges.

3. Meanwhile, line a large baking tray with baking paper. Arrange the sweet potato on the tray, then lightly spray with olive oil and sprinkle with a little paprika. Roast for 20 minutes. Remove the tray from the oven and turn the sweet potato over. Add the onion, sprouts and cauliflower, lightly spray with olive oil and sprinkle with the remaining paprika. Add the garlic cloves, then return the tray to the oven and roast for a further 20 minutes.

4. Squeeze the roasted garlic from the skins and mix with the vinegar and olive oil. Toss through the borlotti beans.

5. Arrange the roasted vegetables on plates and top with the bean mixture. Sprinkle with the thyme, season with freshly ground black pepper and serve.

313 Calories   **42.2 g** Carbs

Nutritional Information

(per serve)

Calories	**313**
Protein	**15.1 g**
Fat Total	**6.8 g**
Fat Saturated	**0.9 g**
Carbohydrates	**42.2 g**
Sugars	**21.6 g**
Sodium	**133.5 mg**
Dietary Fibre	**18.0 g**

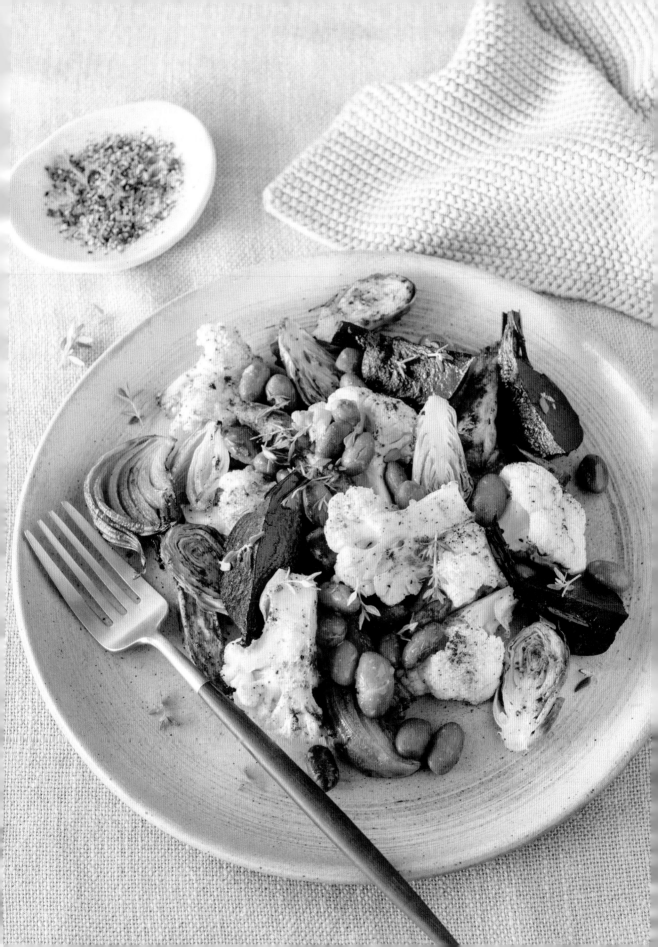

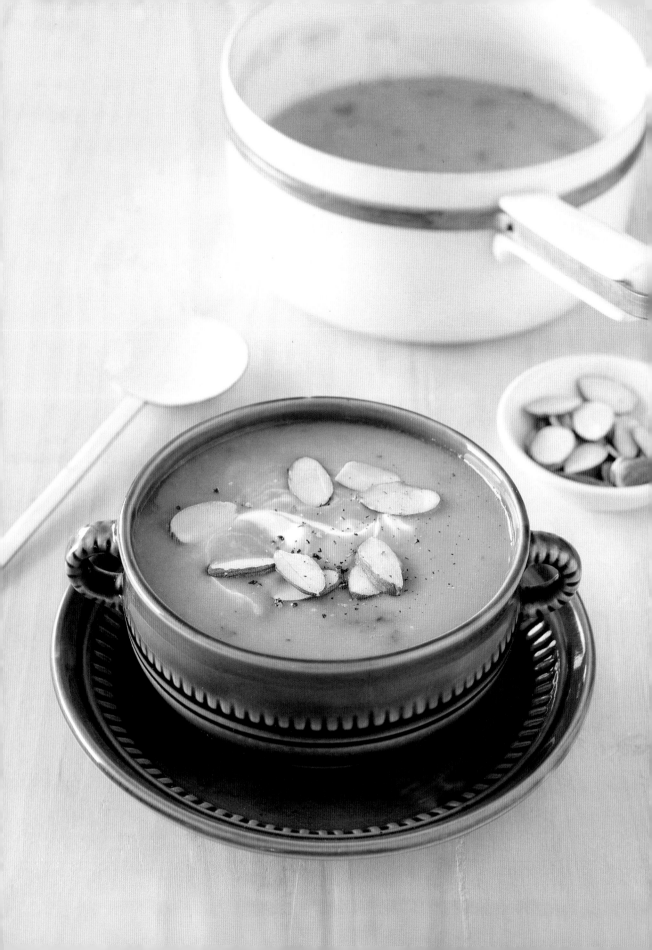

Sweet potato and cannellini bean soup

Sweet potato is the ultimate smart carb and this speedy soup showcases it to perfection.

Serves: **2** • Prep time: **10 minutes** • Cooking time: **10 minutes** • Great for: *Lunch, Dinner or Leftovers*

320	33.7 g
Calories	Carbs

Ingredients

2 teaspoons olive oil

4 spring onions, sliced

2 teaspoons Moroccan seasoning

1 clove garlic, crushed

200 g sweet potato, peeled and chopped

2 cups salt-reduced vegetable stock

1 x 400 g tin cannellini beans, drained and rinsed

1 tablespoon lightly dried coriander

2 tablespoons low-fat natural yoghurt

15 g flaked almonds

Method

1. Heat the olive oil in a saucepan over medium heat. Add the spring onion, Moroccan seasoning and garlic and cook, stirring, for 1 minute. Add the sweet potato and stock. Increase the heat and bring to the boil, then reduce the heat to medium and simmer, partially covered, for 5–8 minutes or until the sweet potato is tender.

2. Stir in the cannellini beans, then remove the pan from the heat and blitz with a hand-held blender until smooth. Return to the heat and warm through. Season with freshly ground black pepper and stir in the coriander. Ladle into bowls and serve topped with the yoghurt and flaked almonds.

Nutritional Information
(per serve)

Calories	**320**
Protein	**14.7 g**
Fat Total	**12.3 g**
Fat Saturated	**1.6 g**
Carbohydrates	**33.7 g**
Sugars	**12.5 g**
Sodium	**1321.7 mg**
Dietary Fibre	**11.7 g**

Mish Tips

Look for 'lightly dried' coriander in the fresh fruit and veg aisle at the supermarket. It has great flavour and colour. Alternatively, sprinkle over some fresh coriander at the end. To reduce the sodium content you can swap the stock for bone broth.

Mushroom and quinoa 'risotto'

Not a quinoa convert yet? This easy recipe is sure to win you over.

Serves: **2** · Prep time: **15 minutes** · Cooking time: **20 minutes** · Great for: *Lunch, Dinner or Leftovers*

Ingredients

2 teaspoons olive oil

½ leek, finely sliced

1 clove garlic, crushed

200 g mushrooms, finely sliced

½ cup salt-reduced vegetable stock

½ cup quinoa, rinsed and drained

80 g baby spinach leaves

3 tablespoons grated parmesan

Method

1. Heat the olive oil in a large saucepan over medium heat, add the leek and garlic and cook, stirring often, for 2 minutes. Add the mushroom and cook, stirring, for 1 minute.

2. Add the stock and quinoa and bring to the boil, then reduce the heat to low and simmer, covered, for 12 minutes. Add the spinach, then cover and simmer for a further 2 minutes.

3. Stir in half the parmesan and season with freshly ground black pepper. Divide between two bowls, sprinkle with the remaining parmesan and serve.

326	35.1 g
Calories	Carbs

Nutritional Information
(per serve)

Calories	**326**
Protein	**16.2 g**
Fat Total	**12.1 g**
Fat Saturated	**3.2 g**
Carbohydrates	**35.1 g**
Sugars	**2.6 g**
Sodium	**439.8 mg**
Dietary Fibre	**6.6 g**

Mish Tips

You can use white, red or black quinoa, or a combination of all three colours.

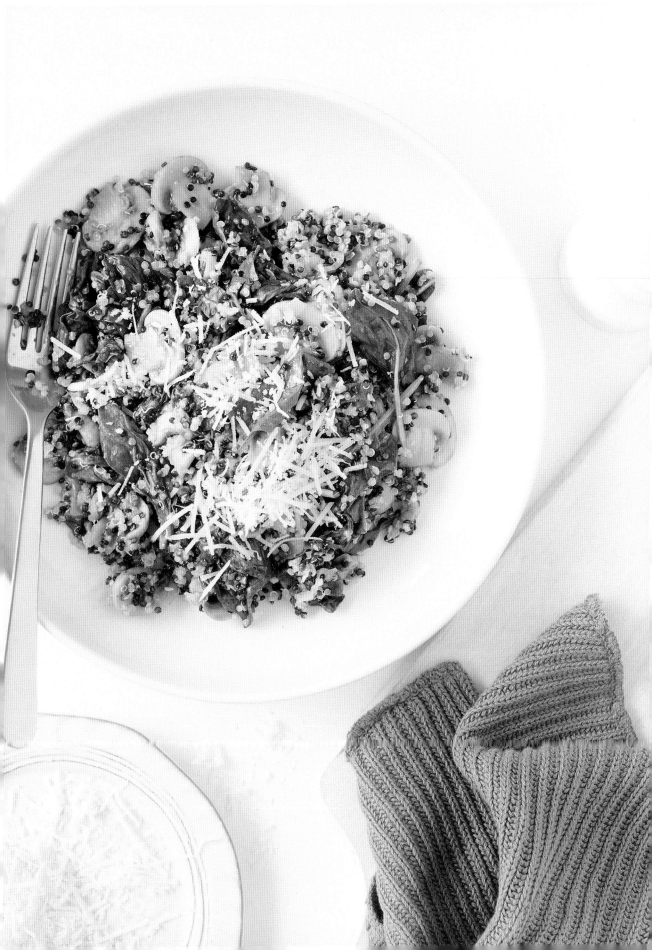

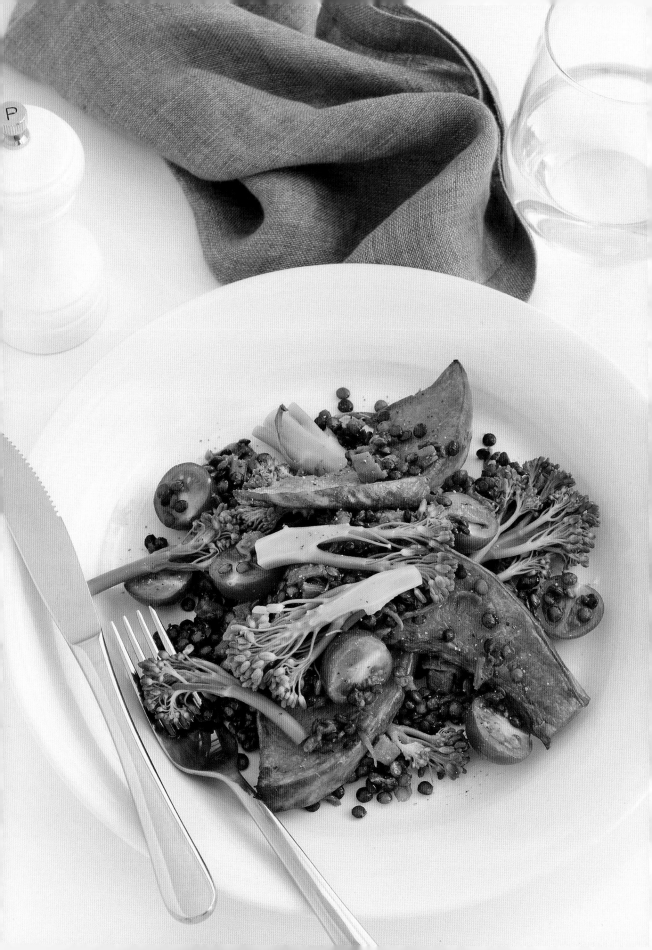

Spiced braised lentils with roasted pumpkin and broccolini

Lentils really are legumes to love! Try this dish on a Meat-free Monday.

Serves: **2** · Prep time: **15 minutes** · Cooking time: **35 minutes** · Great for: *Dinner*

Ingredients

300 g pumpkin, skin left on, cut into wedges

olive oil spray

1 red onion, finely chopped

2 celery stalks, finely chopped

2 cloves garlic, crushed

1 teaspoon ground cumin

1 teaspoon ground coriander

½ cup dried puy-style lentils, rinsed

1 cup salt-reduced vegetable stock

1 bunch broccolini, trimmed

125 g cherry tomatoes, halved

Method

1. Preheat the oven to 200°C (180°C fan-forced). Line a baking tray with baking paper.

2. Place the pumpkin on the prepared tray and lightly spray with olive oil. Roast for 25–30 minutes or until golden and tender.

3. Meanwhile, lightly spray a large saucepan with olive oil and heat over medium heat. Add the onion and celery and cook, stirring occasionally, for 5 minutes or until softened. Add the garlic, cumin and coriander and cook, stirring, for 1 minute or until aromatic.

4. Add the lentils and stock and bring to the boil, then reduce the heat and simmer, partially covered, for 20–25 minutes or until the lentils are tender. Season with freshly ground black pepper.

5. Cook the broccolini in a saucepan of boiling water for 2–3 minutes or until tender. Drain.

6. Serve the braised lentils with the roasted pumpkin, broccolini and cherry tomatoes.

307	**36.3** g
Calories	Carbs

Nutritional Information
(per serve)

Calories	**307**
Protein	**21.7 g**
Fat Total	**3.4 g**
Fat Saturated	**0.4 g**
Carbohydrates	**36.3 g**
Sugars	**17.1 g**
Sodium	**563.0 mg**
Dietary Fibre	**18.6 g**

Mish Tips

Puy-style lentils are green lentils that are slightly smaller than regular brown lentils. They work perfectly here as they hold their shape once cooked. The cooked lentil mixture will keep in an airtight container in the fridge for up to 3 days.

Chargrilled vegetables with crunchy seeds

I love the tastes and textures of this dish. It's truly tempting!

Serves: **2** · Prep time: **20 minutes** · Cooking time: **15 minutes** · Great for: *Lunch, Dinner or Leftovers*

Ingredients

170 g cauliflower, cut into
    bite-sized florets

170 g potato, scrubbed and cut into
    5 mm thick slices

170 g sweet potato, scrubbed and cut
    into 5 mm thick slices

1 zucchini, cut into 2 cm pieces

1 red onion, cut into wedges

olive oil spray

60 g goat's cheese

1 tablespoon crunchy mixed seeds

1 lemon, cut into wedges

Method

1. Preheat a barbecue grill or chargrill pan over medium–high heat. Lightly spray the vegetables with olive oil and season with freshly ground black pepper.

2. Cook the vegetables in two batches for 3–4 minutes each side or until tender and lightly charred.

3. Divide the vegetables between two plates. Crumble over the goat's cheese and scatter with the mixed seeds. Serve with the lemon wedges on the side.

292	31.6 g
Calories	Carbs

Nutritional Information
(per serve)

Calories	**292**
Protein	**14.6 g**
Fat Total	**10.4 g**
Fat Saturated	**4.6 g**
Carbohydrates	**31.6 g**
Sugars	**12.5 g**
Sodium	**140.5 mg**
Dietary Fibre	**10.1 g**

Mish Tips

Crunchy mixed seeds are combinations of sesame, pumpkin, sunflower and sometimes other seeds that have been dry-roasted with soy sauce or tamari. They are available in most supermarkets.

Quinoa, feta, lemon and chilli stuffed capsicum

Quinoa is such a power-packed protein and when it's packed into a roasted capsicum, you can't go wrong!

Serves: **2** · Prep time: **15 minutes** · Cooking time: **45 minutes** · Great for: *Dinner*

320	44.9 g
Calories	Carbs

Ingredients

90 g quinoa, rinsed and drained
olive oil spray
½ red onion, finely chopped
1 clove garlic, crushed
1 small red chilli, seeded and
    finely chopped
2 teaspoons finely grated lemon zest
2 tablespoons chopped
    flat-leaf parsley
40 g low-fat feta, crumbled
20 g currants
1 tomato, chopped
2 red capsicums, halved and seeded
40 g baby rocket leaves

Method

1. Preheat the oven to 200°C (180°C fan-forced). Line a baking tray with baking paper.

2. Cook the quinoa in a saucepan of boiling water for 12 minutes. Drain well and fluff up the grains with a fork.

3. Meanwhile, lightly spray a small non-stick frying pan with olive oil and heat over low heat. Add the onion and cook, stirring occasionally, for 5 minutes or until softened. Add the garlic, chilli and lemon zest and cook, stirring, for 1 minute. Transfer to a bowl and allow to cool slightly.

4. Add the quinoa, parsley, feta, currants and tomato to the bowl, season with freshly ground black pepper and stir to combine. Spoon into the capsicum halves and place on the prepared tray.

5. Cover with foil and bake for 10 minutes. Remove the foil and bake for a further 15–20 minutes or until the capsicums are tender. Serve with the rocket leaves.

Nutritional Information
(per serve)

Calories	**320**
Protein	**15.9 g**
Fat Total	**6.7 g**
Fat Saturated	**4.2 g**
Carbohydrates	**44.9 g**
Sugars	**16.4 g**
Sodium	**256.5 mg**
Dietary Fibre	**9.0 g**

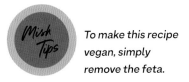

To make this recipe vegan, simply remove the feta.

Chicken and quinoa soup

There is nothing more comforting on a cold winter's day than a bowl of chicken soup, so we have come up with a very easy but tasty recipe that will keep everyone warm and satisfied.

Serves: **2** · Prep time: **15 minutes** · Cooking time: **25 minutes** · Great for: *Lunch, Dinner or Leftovers*

Ingredients

1 teaspoon olive oil
½ leek, halved lengthways and finely sliced
250 g peeled pumpkin, coarsely grated
2 cups salt-reduced chicken stock
200 g lean chicken breast fillet
3 tablespoons quinoa, rinsed and drained
1 carrot, coarsely grated
1 cup shredded Chinese cabbage (wombok)
2 tablespoons chopped flat-leaf parsley

Method

1. Heat the olive oil in a saucepan over medium heat. Add the leek and pumpkin and cook, stirring regularly, for 3 minutes.

2. Pour in the stock and 2 cups water. Cover and bring to a simmer. Add the chicken and cook, partially covered, for 8 minutes. Remove the chicken and set aside on a plate to rest.

3. Add the quinoa to the pan and simmer, covered, for 8 minutes. Add the carrot and cook for a further 3 minutes or until the quinoa is tender.

4. Finely shred the chicken and add to the pan, along with the cabbage. Cook for 1–2 minutes or until the cabbage is tender.

5. Ladle the soup into bowls and season with freshly ground black pepper. Sprinkle with the parsley and serve.

317	**30.2** g
Calories	Carbs

Nutritional Information
(per serve)

Calories	**317**
Protein	**30.7 g**
Fat Total	**6.2 g**
Fat Saturated	**1.3 g**
Carbohydrates	**30.2 g**
Sugars	**13.8 g**
Sodium	**693.4 mg**
Dietary Fibre	**7.5 g**

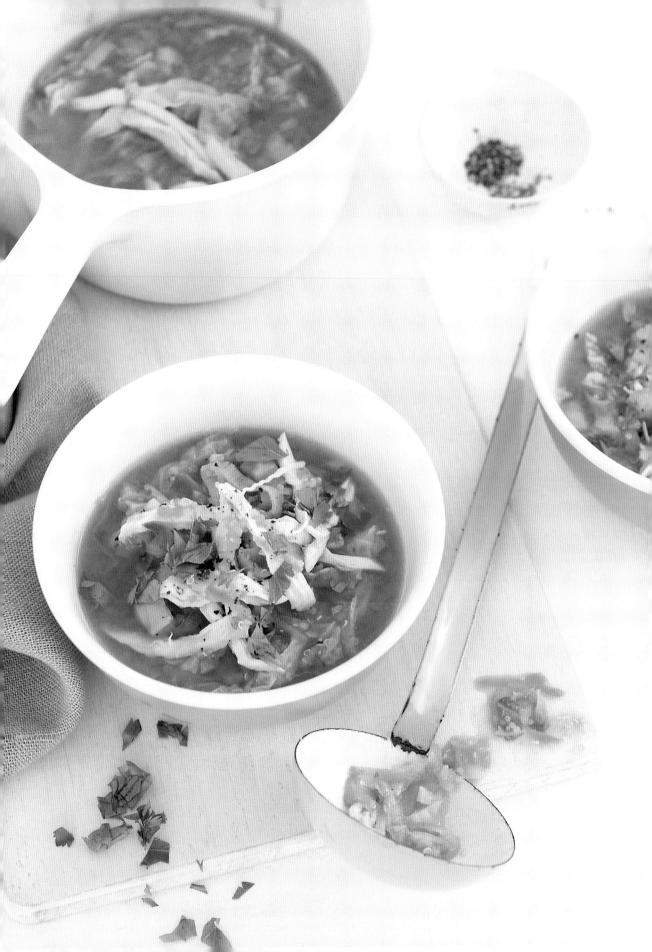

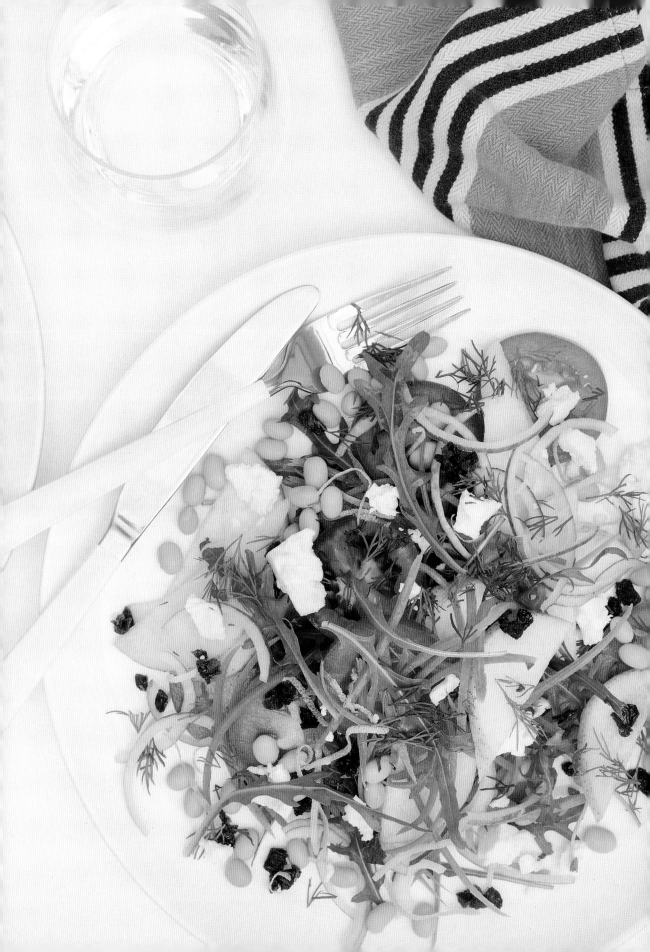

Rocket salad with feta, pear and edamame

A simple rocket salad gets taken to the next level with the addition of edamame and fresh pear. Enjoy!

Serves: **2** · Prep time: **15 minutes** · Great for: *Lunch*

297 **Calories** 38.9 g **Carbs**

Ingredients

80 g thawed, peeled edamame

2 tomatoes, sliced

40 g baby rocket leaves

1 red onion, finely sliced

1 carrot, shredded

1 ripe green pear, halved, cored and finely sliced

50 g raisins, chopped

45 g low-fat feta, crumbled

finely grated zest and juice of 1 lemon

1 tablespoon chopped dill

Method

1. Place the edamame in a heatproof bowl. Cover with boiling water and set aside for 2 minutes. Drain and rinse under cold water.

2. Place the tomato, rocket, onion, carrot, pear, raisins, edamame, feta, lemon zest and dill in a large bowl.

3. Drizzle with half the lemon juice, then add more to taste if you like. Season with freshly ground black pepper and serve.

Nutritional Information

(per serve)

Calories	**297**
Protein	**14.2 g**
Fat Total	**6.0 g**
Fat Saturated	**4.6 g**
Carbohydrates	**38.9 g**
Sugars	**33.6 g**
Sodium	**442.5 mg**
Dietary Fibre	**12.0 g**

Mish Tips

Edamame are fresh soy beans, available from the freezer section of supermarkets and Asian supermarkets. The weight given here is for peeled beans. If you can only buy them in their pods, you will need double the weight to yield the required quantity of beans. If you're making this ahead of time, pack the undressed salad into an airtight container and keep chilled. Dress with the lemon juice just before serving.

Chickpea korma curry

Here we give a classic Indian curry the low-carb
vegetarian treatment. If you'd rather chicken korma,
we've got that for you too — see page 112 for that recipe.

Serves: **2** • Prep time: **15 minutes** • Cooking time: **20 minutes** • Great for: *Lunch, Dinner or Leftovers*

280	33.7 g
Calories	Carbs

Ingredients

olive oil spray

½ brown onion, finely chopped

1 tablespoon korma curry paste

175 g sweet potato, peeled
  and chopped

200 g drained and rinsed
  tinned chickpeas

1½ cups salt-reduced vegetable stock

150 g broccoli, trimmed and cut into
  small florets

75 g green beans, trimmed and sliced

100 g cherry tomatoes, halved

2 tablespoons low-fat natural yoghurt

Method

1. Lightly spray a large saucepan with olive oil
and heat over medium heat. Add the onion and
cook, stirring occasionally, for 5 minutes or until
softened. Add the korma paste and cook, stirring,
for 1 minute or until fragrant.

2. Add the sweet potato, chickpeas and stock and
bring to the boil. Reduce the heat and simmer,
covered, for 10 minutes or until the sweet potato is
almost tender.

3. Add the broccoli, beans and tomatoes and
simmer for a further 3–4 minutes or until the
vegetables are tender.

4. Divide the curry between two bowls and serve
with a dollop of yoghurt on the side.

Nutritional Information

(per serve)

Calories	**280**
Protein	**15.9 g**
Fat Total	**5.6 g**
Fat Saturated	**1.1 g**
Carbohydrates	**33.7 g**
Sugars	**12.8 g**
Sodium	**1108.6 mg**
Dietary Fibre	**13.4 g**

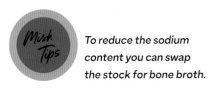

Mish Tips

**To reduce the sodium
content you can swap
the stock for bone broth.**

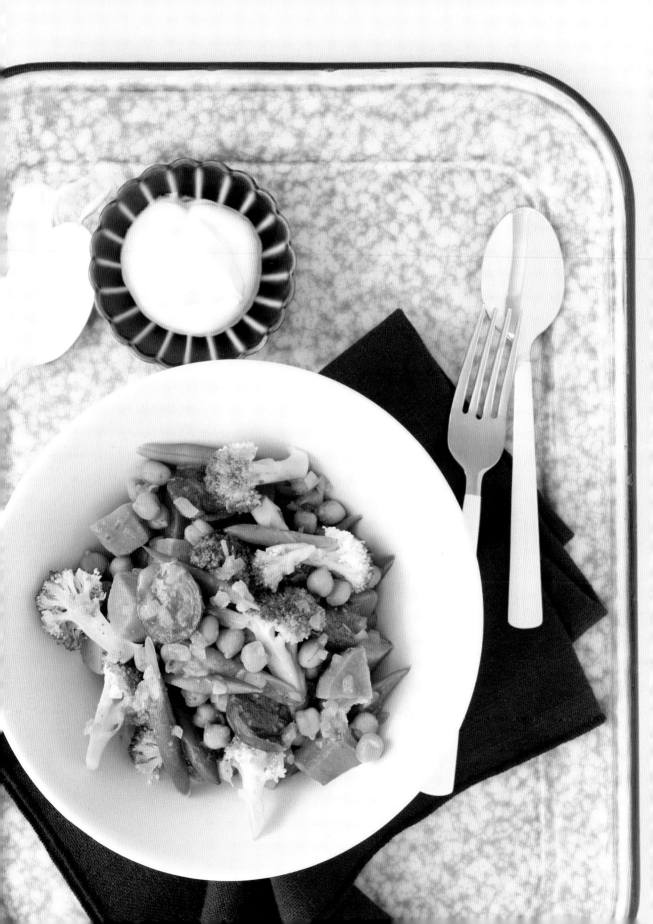

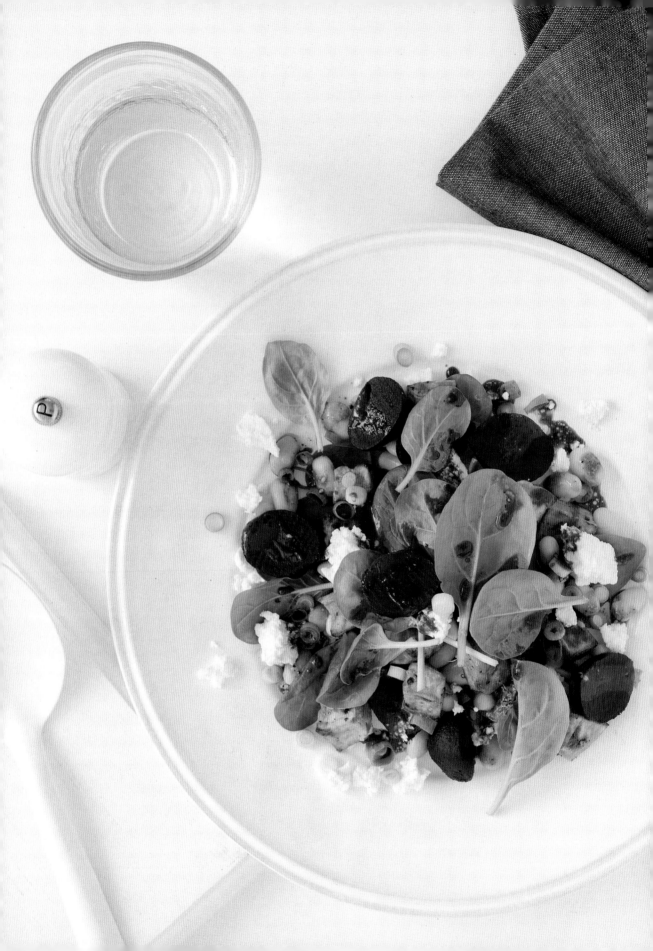

Cannellini bean, beetroot and spinach salad

Cannellini beans are very versatile and lend themselves to many dishes. I love them in this warm salad.

Serves: **2** · Prep time: **15 minutes** · Cooking time: **20 minutes** · Great for: *Weekend Lunch or Dinner*

312	39.7 g
Calories	Carbs

Ingredients

200 g sweet potato, peeled and cut into 1.5 cm cubes

olive oil spray

1 x 400 g tin cannellini beans, drained and rinsed

50 g baby spinach leaves

2 spring onions, sliced

200 g drained tinned beetroot, cut into bite-sized pieces

1 tablespoon balsamic vinegar

1 teaspoon olive oil

1 teaspoon dijon mustard

80 g fresh low-fat ricotta

Method

1. Preheat the oven to 180°C (160°C fan-forced). Line a baking tray with baking paper.

2. Spread out the sweet potato on the prepared tray and lightly spray with olive oil. Bake for 20 minutes or until tender and golden.

3. Meanwhile, place the cannellini beans, spinach, spring onion and beetroot in a bowl and gently combine.

4. Whisk together the balsamic vinegar, olive oil, mustard and freshly ground black pepper in a small bowl. Drizzle the dressing over the salad and toss gently to coat.

5. Divide the salad between plates, crumble the ricotta over the top and serve.

Nutritional Information

(per serve)

Calories	**312**
Protein	**15.5 g**
Fat Total	**7.2 g**
Fat Saturated	**2.9 g**
Carbohydrates	**39.7 g**
Sugars	**18.3 g**
Sodium	**752.8 mg**
Dietary Fibre	**15.0 g**

Chicken with spicy salsa

The star of this dish is the salsa, which features jalapeno chillies. We've used the pickled variety, which are more readily available than fresh, but use what you have to hand. And feel free to add more if you like it hot!

Serves: **2** · Prep time: **15 minutes** · Cooking time: **30 minutes** · Great for: *Dinner*

Ingredients

400 g sweet potato, peeled and cut into half-moon shapes

olive oil spray

250 g lean chicken breast fillet, halved horizontally

1 tomato, diced

1 tablespoon roughly chopped coriander

1 tablespoon roughly chopped flat-leaf parsley

1 tablespoon lime juice

1 spring onion, finely sliced

1 teaspoon finely chopped pickled jalapeno chilli

Method

1. Preheat the oven to 200°C (180°C fan-forced). Line a baking tray with baking paper.

2. Arrange the sweet potato on the prepared tray and lightly spray with olive oil. Bake for 30 minutes or until tender and golden.

3. Meanwhile, lightly spray a non-stick frying pan with olive oil and heat over medium heat. Add the chicken and cook for 3 minutes each side or until golden brown and cooked through.

4. Combine the tomato, coriander, parsley, lime juice, spring onion and chilli in a small bowl.

5. Divide the sweet potato and chicken between plates, top with the salsa and serve.

293	**30.6** g
Calories	Carbs

Nutritional Information

(per serve)

Calories	**293**
Protein	**32.8 g**
Fat Total	**2.9 g**
Fat Saturated	**0.7 g**
Carbohydrates	**30.6 g**
Sugars	**13.4 g**
Sodium	**96.9 mg**
Dietary Fibre	**7.2 g**

You will find pickled jalapeno chillies in the Mexican section of the supermarket.

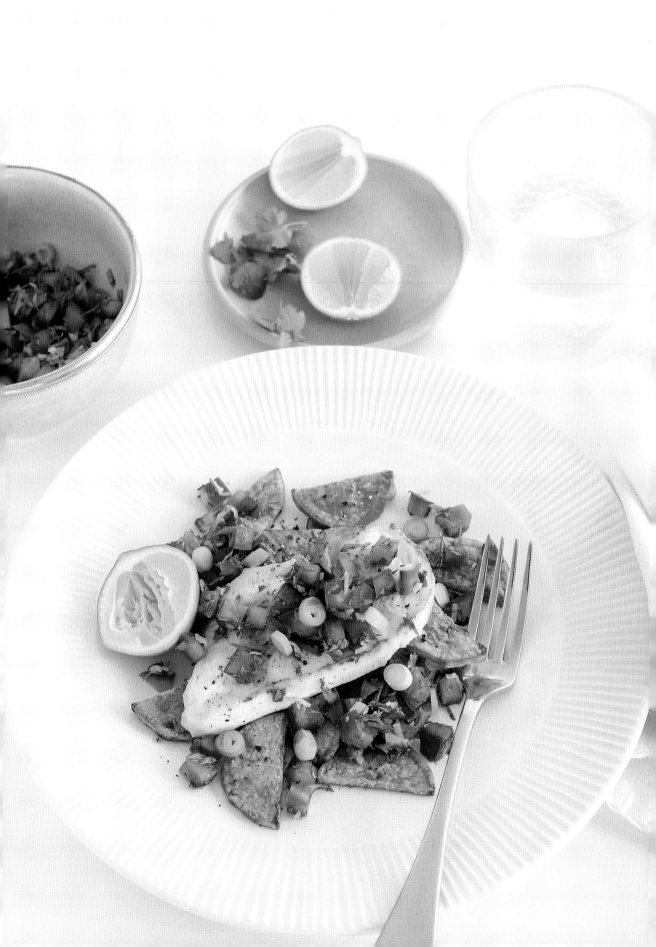

Hearty lentil soup

This wholesome soup makes a simple but very satisfying meal and is very economical. It's easy to double or triple the quantities if need be.

Serves: **2** • Prep time: **10 minutes** • Cooking time: **35 minutes** • Great for: *Lunch, Dinner or Leftovers*

288 **34.7** g
Calories Carbs

Ingredients

olive oil spray
½ brown onion, finely chopped
1 clove garlic, crushed
1 tablespoon tomato paste
1 teaspoon ground cumin
1 teaspoon ground coriander
¾ cup dried red lentils, rinsed
1 carrot, finely chopped
2 cups salt-reduced vegetable stock
2 tablespoons low-fat natural yoghurt
3 tablespoons chopped coriander

Method

1. Lightly spray a saucepan with olive oil and heat over medium heat. Add the onion and garlic and cook, stirring, for 2 minutes or until softened. Add the tomato paste and ground spices and cook, stirring, for 1 minute.

2. Add the lentils, carrot, stock and 3 cups water. Bring to the boil, then reduce the heat to medium–low and simmer, partially covered and stirring occasionally, for 30 minutes or until the lentils and carrot are tender. Season with freshly ground black pepper.

3. Ladle the soup into bowls. Top with a dollop of yoghurt, sprinkle with the chopped coriander and serve.

Nutritional Information

(per serve)

Calories	**288**
Protein	**23.0 g**
Fat Total	**3.7 g**
Fat Saturated	**0.7 g**
Carbohydrates	**34.7 g**
Sugars	**9.1 g**
Sodium	**1051.1 mg**
Dietary Fibre	**13.2 g**

Mish Tips

To reduce the sodium content you can swap the stock for bone broth.

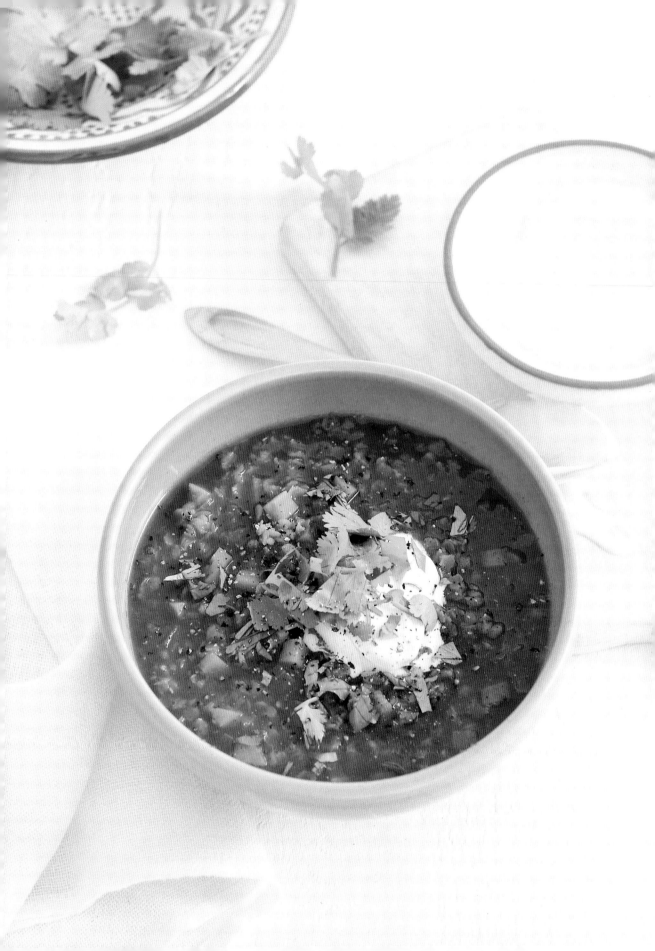

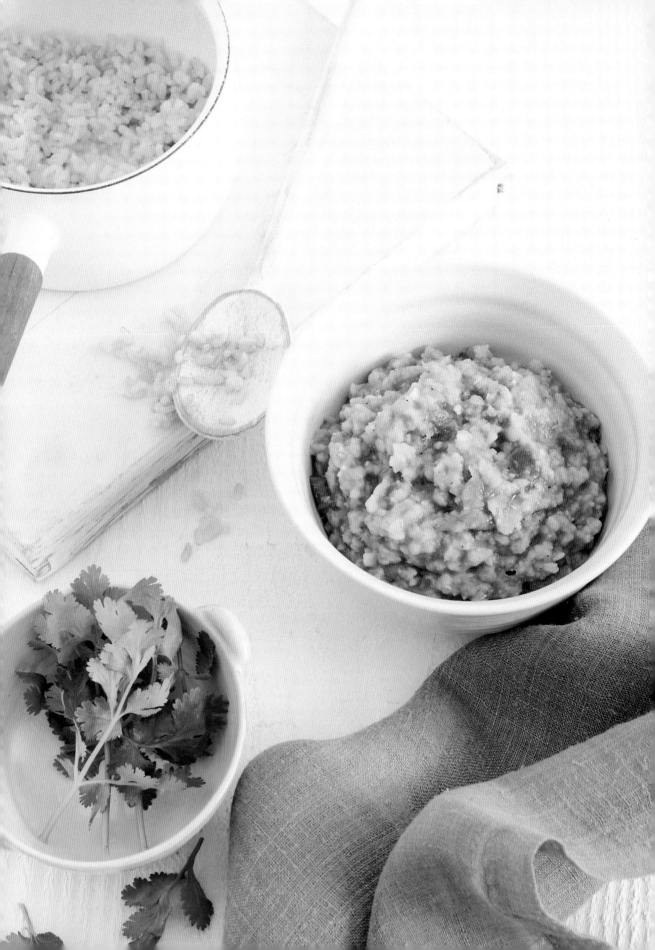

Family dhal

Dhal is delicious, filling and full of nutrition to keep you energised. And this one can be on the table in just half an hour.

Serves: **4** • Prep time: **10 minutes** • Cooking time: **20 minutes** • Great for: *Dinner*

Ingredients

2 cups dried red lentils, rinsed

2 tomatoes, roughly chopped

4 cloves garlic, roughly chopped

1 teaspoon ground cumin

2 teaspoons garam masala

1 teaspoon ground turmeric

1.5 litres salt-reduced vegetable stock

3 tablespoons chopped coriander

Method

1. Combine the lentils, tomato, garlic, cumin, garam masala, turmeric and stock in a large saucepan. Cover and bring to the boil over high heat. Reduce the heat to medium–low and cook, stirring occasionally, for 20 minutes or until the lentils are soft and the dhal has thickened.

2. Ladle the dhal into bowls, sprinkle with the coriander and serve.

330	**39.9** g
Calories	Carbs

Nutritional Information
(per serve)

Calories	**330**
Protein	**26.9 g**
Fat Total	**3.8 g**
Fat Saturated	**0.7 g**
Carbohydrates	**39.9 g**
Sugars	**7.0 g**
Sodium	**1433.9 mg**
Dietary Fibre	**14.8 g**

Feel free to add some chilli if you like your dhal spicy! To reduce the sodium content swap the stock for bone broth. If you need a carb booster, serve the dhal with a side of brown rice.

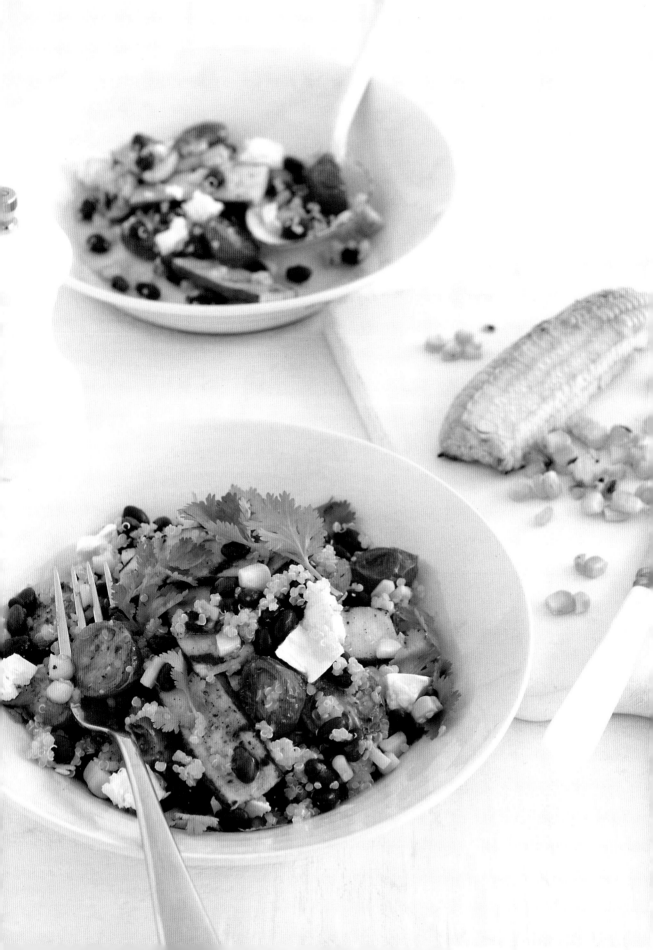

Quinoa salad with roasted corn, black beans and feta

This delicious vegetarian salad features roasted corn, which I absolutely love, and the feta adds a welcome hit of saltiness.

Serves: **2** · Prep time: **20 minutes** · Cooking time: **20 minutes** · Great for: *Lunch*

Ingredients

125 g cherry tomatoes, halved
olive oil spray
⅓ cup quinoa, rinsed and drained
1 corn cob, husk and silks removed
1 zucchini, halved and finely sliced
100 g drained and rinsed tinned black beans
3 tablespoons chopped coriander
1 tablespoon lime juice
1 teaspoon olive oil
40 g low-fat feta, crumbled

Method

1. Preheat the oven to 180°C (160°C fan-forced). Line a large baking tray with baking paper.

2. Place the tomatoes, cut side up, on the prepared tray. Lightly spray with olive oil and season with freshly ground black pepper. Roast for 10 minutes or until just softened. Set aside to cool for 5 minutes.

3. Meanwhile, cook the quinoa in a saucepan of boiling water for 12 minutes. Drain well and fluff up the grains with a fork.

4. Heat a chargrill pan over medium–high heat. Cook the corn, turning occasionally, for 10 minutes or until tender and lightly charred then set aside. Lightly spray the zucchini with olive oil and cook for 2–3 minutes each side or until tender and lightly charred. Set aside to cool slightly. Use a small sharp knife to cut the kernels from the corn cob.

5. Place all the ingredients in a large bowl, season with freshly ground black pepper and gently toss to combine and serve.

336 Calories   **49** g Carbs

Nutritional Information
(per serve)

Calories	**336**
Protein	**17.4 g**
Fat Total	**9.6 g**
Fat Saturated	**4.6 g**
Carbohydrates	**49.0 g**
Sugars	**12.6 g**
Sodium	**237.9 mg**
Dietary Fibre	**11.7 g**

Mish Tips

You can use 1 cup drained tinned corn kernels if you prefer, though the flavour of the roasted corn is delicious. Tinned black beans are different from the Asian variety. Look for them in the Mexican section of your supermarket, or use red kidney beans if you can't find them.

Conversion chart

Measuring cups and spoons may vary slightly from one country to another, but the difference is generally not enough to affect a recipe. All cup and spoon measures are level.
One Australian metric measuring cup holds 250 ml (8 fl oz), one Australian tablespoon holds 20 ml (4 teaspoons) and one Australian metric teaspoon holds 5 ml. North America, New Zealand and the UK use a 15 ml (3-teaspoon) tablespoon.

Length

METRIC	IMPERIAL
3 mm	⅛ inch
6 mm	¼ inch
1 cm	½ inch
2.5 cm	1 inch
5 cm	2 inches
18 cm	7 inches
20 cm	8 inches
23 cm	9 inches
25 cm	10 inches
30 cm	12 inches

Liquid measures

ONE AMERICAN PINT	ONE IMPERIAL PINT
500 ml (16 fl oz)	600 ml (20 fl oz)

CUP	METRIC	IMPERIAL
⅛ cup	30 ml	1 fl oz
¼ cup	60 ml	2 fl oz
⅓ cup	80 ml	2½ fl oz
½ cup	125 ml	4 fl oz
⅔ cup	160 ml	5 fl oz
¾ cup	180 ml	6 fl oz
1 cup	250 ml	8 fl oz
2 cups	500 ml	16 fl oz
2¼ cups	560 ml	20 fl oz
4 cups	1 litre	32 fl oz

Dry measures

The most accurate way to measure dry ingredients is to weigh them. However, if using a cup, add the ingredient loosely to the cup and level with a knife; don't compact the ingredient unless the recipe requests 'firmly packed'.

METRIC	IMPERIAL
15 g	½ oz
30 g	1 oz
60 g	2 oz
125 g	4 oz (¼ lb)
185 g	6 oz
250 g	8 oz (½ lb)
375 g	12 oz (¾ lb)
500 g	16 oz (1 lb)
1 kg	32 oz (2 lb)

Oven temperatures

CELSIUS	FAHRENHEIT
100°C	200°F
120°C	250°F
150°C	300°F
160°C	325°F
180°C	350°F
200°C	400°F
220°C	425°F

CELSIUS	GAS MARK
110°C	¼
130°C	½
140°C	1
150°C	2
170°C	3
180°C	4
190°C	5
200°C	6
220°C	7
230°C	8
240°C	9
250°C	10

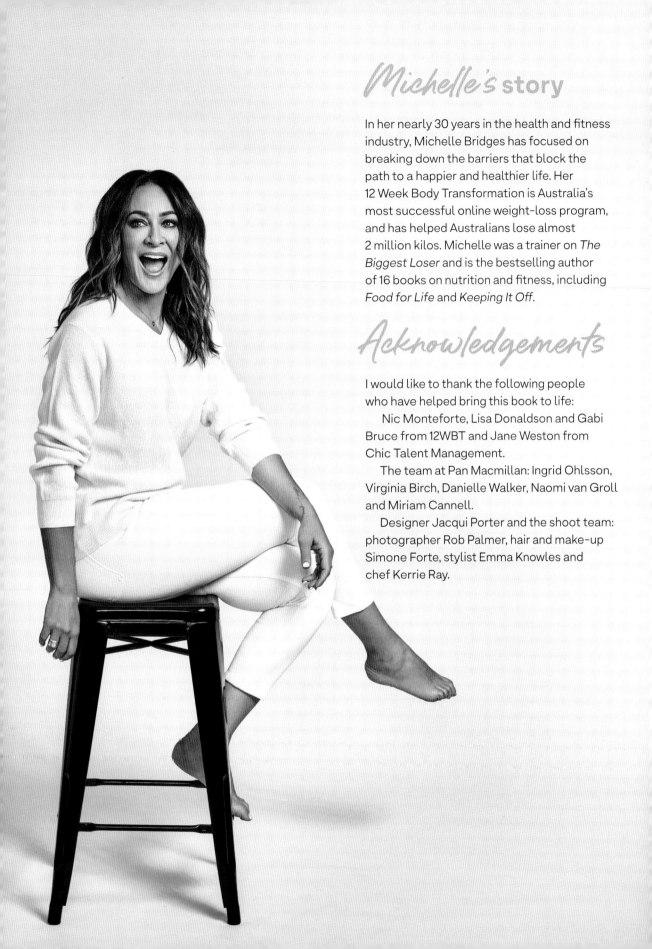

Michelle's story

In her nearly 30 years in the health and fitness industry, Michelle Bridges has focused on breaking down the barriers that block the path to a happier and healthier life. Her 12 Week Body Transformation is Australia's most successful online weight-loss program, and has helped Australians lose almost 2 million kilos. Michelle was a trainer on *The Biggest Loser* and is the bestselling author of 16 books on nutrition and fitness, including *Food for Life* and *Keeping It Off*.

Acknowledgements

I would like to thank the following people who have helped bring this book to life:

Nic Monteforte, Lisa Donaldson and Gabi Bruce from 12WBT and Jane Weston from Chic Talent Management.

The team at Pan Macmillan: Ingrid Ohlsson, Virginia Birch, Danielle Walker, Naomi van Groll and Miriam Cannell.

Designer Jacqui Porter and the shoot team: photographer Rob Palmer, hair and make-up Simone Forte, stylist Emma Knowles and chef Kerrie Ray.

Index

A
Asian chicken omelette 73
asparagus
Carrot and asparagus noodles with coriander and coconut dressing 146
Hoisin beef stir-fry with spring vegetables 150
Warm chicken salad 70
Warm potato salad with prawns and asparagus 128
avocados
Kale, macadamia and tomato salad with avocado 142
Roasted capsicum and ham frittata with avocado and herb salad 77
Salmon, avocado and walnut salad 98
Scrambled eggs with spinach and avocado 95
Smoked tofu, pickled ginger, avocado and quinoa sushi 186
Super green smoothie 213

B
Baba ganoush 39
Baked mushrooms 120
Balsamic and basil strawberries with ricotta 42
Barbecued steak with iceberg lettuce 121
beans
Beef and bean soup 208
Beef and mushrooms with mash 123
Beetroot salad with smoked tofu and beans 200
Cannellini bean, beetroot and spinach salad 243
Celeriac and white bean soup 176
Italian turkey meatball tray bake 167
Quinoa and kidney bean chilli 222
Quinoa salad with roasted corn, black beans and feta 251
Rainbow salad jar 172
Roasted mushrooms with honey soy sweet potato 225
Salmon and edamame salad 127
Sweet potato and cannellini bean soup 229
Sweet potato and tuna poke bowl 170
Tomato fish stew 137
Warm winter vegetable salad 226
see also green beans
beef
Baked mushrooms 120
Barbecued steak with iceberg lettuce 121
Beef and bean soup 208
Beef and mushrooms with mash 123
Hoisin beef stir-fry with spring vegetables 150
Low-FODMAP steak with grilled summer veggies 155
Mexican cottage pie 181
Peppered steak with mashed peas and roasted cherry tomatoes 189
Roast beef dinner 180
Steak with creamy mushroom sauce 92
Warm Mediterranean beef salad 108
beetroot
Beetroot salad with smoked tofu and beans 200
Buddha bowl 218
Cannellini bean, beetroot and spinach salad 243
Dukkah-crusted pork with roasted vegetable salad 183
Grated beetroot and chickpea fritters 104
Lamb with beetroot puree and herbed peas 149
Rainbow salad jar 172
Rainbow vegetable salad 139
Warm winter vegetable salad 226

Braised pumpkin and lentils with haloumi 168
breakfast recipe index 61
broccoli
Chicken and vegetables in coconut 154
Chickpea korma curry 240
Grilled fish with herbed veggie 'couscous' 74
Pork with sweet potato chips and broccoli salad 202
Raw broccoli and lentil salad 204
Spicy chicken and broccoli stir-fry 145
Veggie and tofu tray bake with feta cream 68
broccolini
Beef and mushrooms with mash 123
Hoisin beef stir-fry with spring vegetables 150
Kangaroo with mint yoghurt and pea salad 132
Lamb steaks with spiced sweet potato and coriander mash 184
Pork meatballs with fennel and apple slaw 107
Salmon and edamame salad 127
Spiced braised lentils with roasted pumpkin and broccolini 233
Steak with creamy mushroom sauce 92
Veal goulash 179
Buddha bowl 218

C
Cacao fudge bites 42
Cannellini bean, beetroot and spinach salad 243
capsicum
Asian chicken omelette 73
Capsicum and cottage cheese 40
Capsicum and hummus 41
Charred chicken, corn and mango salad 194
Chicken and lettuce 'tacos' 116
Low-FODMAP steak with grilled summer veggies 155
Portuguese piri piri chicken with quinoa salad 164
Potato, spinach and feta tortilla 152
Quinoa, feta, lemon and chilli stuffed capsicum 235
Rainbow vegetable salad 139
Roasted capsicum and ham frittata with avocado and herb salad 77
Roasted vegetable frittata 191
Spicy chicken and broccoli stir-fry 145
Tuna frittata 169
Turkey meatballs in tomato sauce 124
Warm Mediterranean beef salad 108
carbohydrates 12–15
and gut health 18–19
balancing with protein and fat 22–3
carb boosters 45
choosing 21
low-carb eating 20
my favourite smart carbs 24–5
quality carbs 21
simple and complex 12
simple carb swaps 26–7
carrots
Carrot and asparagus noodles with coriander and coconut dressing 146
Chicken and vegetables in coconut 154
Chicken curry patties with veggie noodles 64
Ginger and lemongrass roast chicken 110
Hearty lentil soup 246
Lamb with Moroccan carrot salad 156
Mexican cottage pie 181
Roast beef dinner 180
Rocket salad with feta, pear and edamame 239
Seared salmon with vegetable noodles 90
Steak with creamy mushroom sauce 92
Veggie and tofu tray bake with feta cream 68
case study: Nerida's story 31

cauliflower
Buddha bowl 218
Chargrilled vegetables with crunchy seeds 234
Chicken and vegetables in coconut 154
Ginger and lemongrass roast chicken 110
Miso cauliflower bites 39
Miso salmon with cauliflower fried rice 66
Veggie and tofu tray bake with feta cream 68
Warm winter vegetable salad 226
Celeriac and white bean soup 176
Chargrilled vegetables with crunchy seeds 234
Charred chicken, corn and mango salad 194
chicken
Asian chicken omelette 73
Charred chicken, corn and mango salad 194
Chicken and lettuce 'tacos' 116
Chicken and quinoa soup 236
Chicken and vegetables in coconut 154
Chicken curry patties with veggie noodles 64
Chicken kebabs with radish and cucumber salad 80
Chicken with spicy salsa 244
Chicken, lentil and kale soup 134
Chicken, pumpkin and chickpeas 113
Ginger and lemongrass roast chicken 110
Mild chicken korma 112
Portuguese piri piri chicken with quinoa salad 164
Prosciutto-wrapped chicken with wilted greens 82
Spicy chicken and broccoli stir-fry 145
Summery lemon, honey and rosemary chicken 198
Warm chicken salad 70
chickpeas 25
Chicken and vegetables in coconut 154
Chicken, pumpkin and chickpeas 113
Chickpea korma curry 240
Crunchy spiced chickpeas 38
Ginger and lemongrass roast chicken 110
Grated beetroot and chickpea fritters 104
Lamb with Moroccan carrot salad 156
conversion chart 252
cravings 37
Crunchy spiced chickpeas 38
cucumber
Barbecued steak with iceberg lettuce 121
Chicken kebabs with radish and cucumber salad 80
Portuguese piri piri chicken with quinoa salad 164
Roast lamb with lemon, garlic and rosemary 140
Smoked tofu, pickled ginger, avocado and quinoa sushi 186
Thai fish cakes with bean sprout salad 96
Warm lamb, pumpkin and pomegranate salad with minty yoghurt dressing 175

D
diabetes 14, 15, 16, 17
Dukkah-crusted pork with roasted vegetable salad 183

E
eating out 29
eggplant
Baba ganoush 39
Eggplant, sweet potato and ricotta bake 173
Low-FODMAP pumpkin and spinach lasagne 144
Roasted vegetable frittata 191
Sweet potato, mushroom and feta stacks 206
Warm lamb, pumpkin and pomegranate salad with minty yoghurt dressing 175
eggs
Asian chicken omelette 73
Beetroot salad with smoked tofu and beans 200
Egg-power! 41

Italian-style baked eggs 85
Japanese tofu and cabbage pancake 88
Lentil salad with poached eggs 114
Mushroom omelettes with spinach and cherry tomatoes 81
Potato, spinach and feta tortilla 152
Roasted capsicum and ham frittata with avocado and herb salad 77
Roasted vegetable frittata 191
Salmon nicoise salad 129
Scrambled eggs with spinach and avocado 95
Souffle omelette with spinach and mushrooms 99
Tuna frittata 169
Zucchini and herb frittata 192
exercise 17, 32–5

F
Family dhal 249
fasting and low-carb eating 29
fatty liver 16
fibre 18–19
fish
Fish kebabs with green leaf salad 78
Grilled fish with herbed veggie 'couscous' 74
Thai fish cakes with bean sprout salad 96
Tomato fish stew 137
see also salmon, tuna
flour, refined white 15
fructose 16

G
Garlic and thyme grilled mushrooms 38
Ginger and lemongrass roast chicken 110
Grated beetroot and chickpea fritters 104
green beans
Chickpea korma curry 240
Italian turkey meatball tray bake 167
Mild chicken korma 112
Quick prawn curry 89
Salmon nicoise salad 129
Summery lemon, honey and rosemary chicken 198
Warm chicken salad 70
Grilled fish with herbed veggie 'couscous' 74
gut–brain connection 19

H
haloumi
Braised pumpkin and lentils with haloumi 168
Smoky vegetable and haloumi kebabs with lemony rocket salad 130
Hearty lentil soup 246
Hoisin beef stir-fry with spring vegetables 150

I
ingredient swaps 26–7, 46–7
insulin resistance 14, 16
Italian turkey meatball tray bake 167
Italian-style baked eggs 85

J
Japanese tofu and cabbage pancake 88

K
Kale, macadamia and tomato salad with avocado 142
Kangaroo with mint yoghurt and pea salad 132
keto diet 20

L
lamb
Lamb slaw 118
Lamb steaks with spiced sweet potato and coriander mash 184
Lamb with beetroot puree and herbed peas 149
Lamb with Moroccan carrot salad 156
Oven-roasted lamb rack with tomatoes and salsa verde 86
Roast lamb with lemon, garlic and rosemary 140
Warm lamb, pumpkin and pomegranate salad with minty yoghurt dressing 175
leftovers, how to use 61

12WBT Low-carb Solution

lentils 24
  Braised pumpkin and lentils with haloumi 168
  Chicken, lentil and kale soup 134
  Family dhal 249
  Hearty lentil soup 246
  Lentil salad with poached eggs 114
  Low-FODMAP pumpkin and spinach lasagne 144
  Raw broccoli and lentil salad 204
  Spiced braised lentils with roasted pumpkin and broccolini 233
  Zucchini noodles with lentils and feta 103
liver, fatty 16
Low-FODMAP pumpkin and spinach lasagne 144
Low-FODMAP steak with grilled summer veggies 155

M
mangos
  Charred chicken, corn and mango salad 194
  Summer smoothie bowl 214
  Tropical fruit salad with toasted coconut yoghurt 216
meal plans 45, 48–57
metabolic syndrome 16, 17
Mexican cottage pie 181
Mild chicken korma 112
Mini tomato, bocconcini and basil skewers 40
Miso cauliflower bites 39
Miso salmon with cauliflower fried rice 66
mushrooms
  Baked mushrooms 120
  Beef and mushrooms with mash 123
  Braised pumpkin and lentils with haloumi 168
  Eggplant, sweet potato and ricotta bake 173
  Garlic and thyme grilled mushrooms 38
  Mushroom and quinoa 'risotto' 230
  Mushroom omelettes with spinach and cherry tomatoes 81
  Roasted mushrooms with honey soy sweet potato 225
  Smoky vegetable and haloumi kebabs with lemony rocket salad 130
  Souffle omelette with spinach and mushrooms 99
  Steak with creamy mushroom sauce 92
  Sweet potato, mushroom and feta stacks 206
  Tofu and greens stir-fry 196
  Veal goulash 179
my day on a plate 28–9

N
nutritional information 60

O
obesity 15
Oven-roasted lamb rack with tomatoes and salsa verde 86

P
Papaya with lime and coconut cream 43
Peppered steak with mashed peas and roasted cherry tomatoes 189
pineapple
  Pineapple carpaccio with ginger and mint yoghurt 43
  Pork with grilled pineapple 221
  Super green smoothie 213
  Tropical fruit salad with toasted coconut yoghurt 216
pork
  Dukkah-crusted pork with roasted vegetable salad 183
  Pork meatballs with fennel and apple slaw 107
  Pork with grape and cabbage salad 136
  Pork with grilled pineapple 221
  Pork with sweet potato chips and broccoli salad 202
  Prosciutto-wrapped chicken with wilted greens 82
  Roasted capsicum and ham frittata with avocado and herb salad 77

Portuguese piri piri chicken with quinoa salad 164
potatoes 25
  Chargrilled vegetables with crunchy seeds 234
  Italian turkey meatball tray bake 167
  Potato, spinach and feta tortilla 152
  Salmon nicoise salad 129
  Salmon, avocado and walnut salad 98
  Summery lemon, honey and rosemary chicken 198
  Veal goulash 179
  Warm potato salad with prawns and asparagus 128
  Zucchini and herb frittata 192
prawns
  Prawn parcels 38
  Quick prawn curry 89
  Saganaki-style prawns 162
  Warm potato salad with prawns and asparagus 128
prebiotic foods 18
probiotic foods 18
Prosciutto-wrapped chicken with wilted greens 82
pumpkin
  Braised pumpkin and lentils with haloumi 168
  Buddha bowl 218
  Chicken and quinoa soup 236
  Chicken, pumpkin and chickpeas 113
  Low-FODMAP pumpkin and spinach lasagne 144
  Spiced braised lentils with roasted pumpkin and broccolini 233
  Warm lamb, pumpkin and pomegranate salad with minty yoghurt dressing 175

Q
Quick prawn curry 89
quinoa
  Buddha bowl 218
  Chicken and quinoa soup 236
  Mushroom and quinoa 'risotto' 230
  Portuguese piri piri chicken with quinoa salad 164
  Quinoa and kidney bean chilli 222
  Quinoa salad with roasted corn, black beans and feta 251
  Quinoa, feta, lemon and chilli stuffed capsicum 235
  Smoked tofu, pickled ginger, avocado and quinoa sushi 186
  Tofu and greens stir-fry 196

R
Rainbow salad jar 172
Rainbow vegetable salad 139
Raw broccoli and lentil salad 204
recipes, navigating 60–1
Roast beef dinner 180
Roast lamb with lemon, garlic and rosemary 140
Roasted capsicum and ham frittata with avocado and herb salad 77
Roasted mushrooms with honey soy sweet potato 225
Roasted vegetable frittata 191
Rocket salad with feta, pear and edamame 239

S
Saganaki-style prawns 162
salmon
  Fish kebabs with green leaf salad 78
  Miso salmon with cauliflower fried rice 66
  Salmon and edamame salad 127
  Salmon, avocado and walnut salad 98
  Salmon nicoise salad 129
  Scrambled eggs with spinach and avocado 95
  Seared salmon with vegetable noodles 90
  Smoked tofu, pickled ginger, avocado and quinoa sushi 186
  Smoky vegetable and haloumi kebabs with lemony rocket salad 130
Snack balls 43

snacks
  savoury 38–9
  speedy 40–1
  sweet 42–3
Souffle omelette with spinach and mushrooms 99
Spiced braised lentils with roasted pumpkin and broccolini 233
Spicy chicken and broccoli stir-fry 145
starch, resistant 19
Steak with creamy mushroom sauce 92
strawberries
  Balsamic and basil strawberries with ricotta 42
  Strawberry ballerinas 41
  Sweet spiced yoghurt dip with strawberries 42
sugar 12, 14–15
Summer smoothie bowl 214
Summery lemon, honey and rosemary chicken 198
Super green smoothie 213
sweet potatoes 24
  Beef and mushrooms with mash 123
  Cannellini bean, beetroot and spinach salad 243
  Chargrilled vegetables with crunchy seeds 234
  Chicken with spicy salsa 244
  Chickpea korma curry 240
  Dukkah-crusted pork with roasted vegetable salad 183
  Eggplant, sweet potato and ricotta bake 173
  Lamb steaks with spiced sweet potato and coriander mash 184
  Low-FODMAP steak with grilled summer veggies 155
  Mexican cottage pie 181
  Mild chicken korma 112
  Peppered steak with mashed peas and roasted cherry tomatoes 189
  Pork with grilled pineapple 221
  Pork with sweet potato chips and broccoli salad 202
  Roast beef dinner 180
  Roast lamb with lemon, garlic and rosemary 140
  Roasted mushrooms with honey soy sweet potato 225
  Roasted vegetable frittata 191
  Sweet potato and cannellini bean soup 229
  Sweet potato and tuna poke bowl 170
  Sweet potato, mushroom and feta stacks 206
  Sweet spiced yoghurt dip with strawberries 42
  Warm winter vegetable salad 226

T
Thai fish cakes with bean sprout salad 96
Tinned tuna 41
tofu
  Beetroot salad with smoked tofu and beans 200
  Japanese tofu and cabbage pancake 88
  Smoked tofu, pickled ginger, avocado and quinoa sushi 186
  Tofu and greens stir-fry 196
  Veggie and tofu tray bake with feta cream 68
tomatoes
  Chicken and lettuce 'tacos' 116
  Chicken with spicy salsa 244
  Chickpea korma curry 240
  Family dhal 249
  Italian turkey meatball tray bake 167
  Italian-style baked eggs 85
  Kale, macadamia and tomato salad with avocado 142
  Low-FODMAP steak with grilled summer veggies 155
  Mini tomato, bocconcini and basil skewers 40
  Mushroom omelettes with spinach and cherry tomatoes 81
  Oven-roasted lamb rack with tomatoes and salsa verde 86

Peppered steak with mashed peas and roasted cherry tomatoes 189
Quinoa salad with roasted corn, black beans and feta 251
Quinoa, feta, lemon and chilli stuffed capsicum 235
Rainbow salad jar 172
Raw broccoli and lentil salad 204
Roast lamb with lemon, garlic and rosemary 140
Roasted mushrooms with honey soy sweet potato 225
Rocket salad with feta, pear and edamame 239
Salmon nicoise salad 129
Scrambled eggs with spinach and avocado 95
Spiced braised lentils with roasted pumpkin and broccolini 233
Sweet potato and tuna poke bowl 170
Tomato fish stew 137
Tuna frittata 169
Turkey meatballs in tomato sauce 124
Warm Mediterranean beef salad 108
Zucchini and herb frittata 192
Zucchini cakes with dill raita 158
Zucchini noodles with lentils and feta 103
Tropical fruit salad with toasted coconut yoghurt 216
tuna
  Rainbow vegetable salad 139
  Sweet potato and tuna poke bowl 170
  Tinned tuna 41
  Tuna frittata 169
turkey
  Italian turkey meatball tray bake 167
  Turkey meatballs in tomato sauce 124

V
Veal goulash 179
Veggie and tofu tray bake with feta cream 68
Veggie sticks with hummus 40

W
Warm chicken salad 70
Warm lamb, pumpkin and pomegranate salad with minty yoghurt dressing 175
Warm Mediterranean beef salad 108
Warm potato salad with prawns and asparagus 128
Warm winter vegetable salad 226
workouts 33–5

Z
zucchini
  Baked mushrooms 120
  Beef and bean soup 208
  Chargrilled vegetables with crunchy seeds 234
  Chicken curry patties with veggie noodles 64
  Ginger and lemongrass roast chicken 110
  Grilled fish with herbed veggie 'couscous' 74
  Italian-style baked eggs 85
  Kale, macadamia and tomato salad with avocado 142
  Low-FODMAP pumpkin and spinach lasagne 144
  Low-FODMAP steak with grilled summer veggies 155
  Mexican cottage pie 181
  Quick prawn curry 89
  Quinoa and kidney bean chilli 222
  Quinoa salad with roasted corn, black beans and feta 251
  Seared salmon with vegetable noodles 90
  Smoky vegetable and haloumi kebabs with lemony rocket salad 130
  Tomato fish stew 137
  Tuna frittata 169
  Turkey meatballs in tomato sauce 124
  Warm Mediterranean beef salad 108
  Zucchini and herb frittata 192
  Zucchini cakes with dill raita 158
  Zucchini noodles with lentils and feta 103

First published 2020 in Macmillan
by Pan Macmillan Australia Pty Limited
Level 25, 1 Market Street, Sydney, New South Wales
Australia 2000

A CIP catalogue record for this book is available from the National Library of Australia:
http://catalogue.nla.gov.au

Design by Northwood Green
Edited by Miriam Cannell
Recipe editing by Rachel Carter
Index by Helena Holmgren
Prop and food styling by Emma Knowles (for pages 2–3,
    13, 16, 17, 24–27, 30, 36, 37: bottom left, 38–44, 46–47, 56–57)
Food preparation by Kerrie Ray (for pages 2–3, 13, 16, 17,
    24–27, 30, 36, 37: bottom left, 38–44, 46–47, 56–57)
Hair and make-up by Simone Forte
Colour + reproduction by Splitting Image Colour Studio
Printed and bound in China by Imago Printing International Limited

10 9 8 7 6 5 4 3 2 1